Bodybuilding For Beginners

STRONGER
THAN EVER!

Transform Your Body Into A
Fighting Machine

Brent Green

Chapter 1: Setting Yourself Up For Success

How Your Diet Affects Your Results

Exercise and diet are equally important factors to building muscle and losing fat. It is generally touted that diet may even play a larger role in the outcome of your fitness. If you are working out hard and not seeing results, make sure that the things you are eating are unprocessed and have high nutrient values—more specifically, work with a nutritionist to find the macronutrient intake levels that are right for the goal you are trying to reach.

Warm Up Before Working Out

To avoid injury, we should take some time before starting our workout to warm up all of our muscle groups. It is generally accepted that warming up before a workout will lead to better performance results and decrease the chance of injuring yourself. Don't forget to stretch after you're done, too! Warming up and cooling down should take no less than 5 minutes, but no more than 15-20 minutes. We don't want all your time spent prepping for your workout or stretching afterward, but they are important components that ensure your body's continued functionality.

Example Warm Up Workouts:

Complete these exercises for 5-10 minutes

1. Jog, row, or ride a bike at a slow-medium pace

2. Jump rope

3. High knees or butt kicks

4. Walk-out planks

5. Jumping jacks

Important Areas to Stretch:

Areas are followed by examples

1. Arms: arm circles

2. Legs: walking lunges

3. Glutes: glute bridge

4. Calves: wall lean

5. Back: leg pull

When warming up, we want our heart rate to increase, so make sure that while you are completing these exercises, you are adequately exerting yourself. We want our body to be ready for the more intense activity we are about to take part in. An increase in blood flow, an increase in body temperature, and an increase in breathing rate all build slowly through warming up in preparation. If you need to ask yourself if you are working out vigorously enough, a good test to check is to see if you would be able to keep a conversation going with your friend. If you are working out hard enough, you really shouldn't be able to keep a conversation going.

Who These Workouts Are Best-Suited For

Bodyweight Workouts are best-suited for those who cannot afford a gym membership, don't enjoy the gym atmosphere, or for those who feel like they are too large to jump right into fast-paced routines. Memberships can be expensive depending on where you go, and we don't all have enough money to afford one at certain points in our lives. Many people—women, in particular—feel uncomfortable at the gym or are intimidated by the size of the facility and the variety of equipment. Bodyweight Workouts can be modified for someone of any shape and size and can be completed in the privacy of your own home if you are self-conscious by working out in public.

Benefits of Bodyweight Workouts

These workouts allow you to build muscle, gain strength, and increase your stamina by using nothing other than your body. Able to be completed anywhere and with no equipment, Bodyweight Workouts are fast and effective. The Huffington Post contributor Dave Smith lists the numerous benefits of Bodyweight Workouts:

1. They are efficient: "Research suggests high-output, bodyweight-based exercises such as plyometrics yield awesome fitness gains in very short workout durations. Since there's no equipment involved, bodyweight workouts make it easy to transition quickly from one exercise to the next. Shorter rest times mean it's easy to boost heart rate and burn some serious calories quickly."

2. There's something for everyone: "Bodyweight exercises are a great choice because they're easily modified to challenge any fitness level. Adding extra repetitions, performing the exercises faster or super-slow, and perfecting form are a few ways to make even the simplest exercise more challenging. And progress is easy to measure since bodyweight exercises offer endless ways to do a little more in each workout."

3. They can improve core strength: "The 'core' is not just the abs. At least 29 muscles make up our core. Many bodyweight movements can be used to engage all of them. These will improve core strength, resulting in better posture and improved athletic performance."

4. <u>Workouts are convenient</u>: "Ask someone why they don't exercise. Chances are they'll answer they have 'no time' or that it's an 'inconvenience.' These common obstacles are eliminated by bodyweight exercises because they allow anyone to squeeze in workouts any time, anywhere. It can be a stress reliever for those who work at home, or it can be a great hotel room workout for people on the road. With bodyweight workouts, 'no time' becomes no excuse."

5. <u>Workouts can be fun and easily mixed up for variety</u>: "It can be easy to get stuck in a workout rut of bench presses, lat pull-downs, and biceps curls. That's why bodyweight training can be so refreshing: There are countless exercise variations that can spice up any workout routine. Working with a variety of exercises not only relieves potential workout boredom, but it can also help break through exercise plateaus to spark further fitness progress."

6. <u>They can provide quick results</u>: "Bodyweight exercises get results partly because they often involve compound movements. Compound exercises such as push-ups, lunges, and chin-ups have been shown to be extremely effective for strength gains and performance improvements."

Creating a Workout Environment

Since these workouts can be complete at home, making sure you have available space to complete exercises is imperative for success. All you really need is a space large enough to spread out a little bit—let's say for example, to complete 10 lunges in a row. While you do not need any equipment, it may be nice to have a yoga mat if you have hard floors like wood or linoleum.

Some prefer a quiet environment to work out or to use a music player to help them focus during their workout. Do whatever puts you in the zone to complete your routine. The point is to try to minimize the space of distractions so you can put in the work to meet your goals.

Summary and Key Points

Bodyweight Workouts are easy, fast, and are extremely effective for beginners and more seasoned exercisers!

You can't expect the most comprehensive results without also ensuring your diet falls in line with the changes you want to see on your body!

Designate a space to complete your workouts in, whether that be your living room or backyard patio.

Design your space to allow for workout completion depending on space needs and create motivational vibes in the area for inspiration.

Chapter 2: Types of Bodyweight Workouts

Bodyweight workouts can be focused on targeting a specific group of muscles. This chapter will outline bodyweight exercises that target the following areas: arms, legs, chest, back, butt, and abs.

We all have what we call 'problem areas,' and strength training can be the best and fastest way to target those areas on our bodies that we want to be more toned. Bodyweight Workouts use our own weight to create resistance so we can work on building up muscle on whichever body parts need our attention. Here are some examples of workouts from the before-named areas:

Focus: Arms

Tricep Dips

- o This move helps build up your pectorals, triceps, forearms, and shoulder muscles. Push your chest out and using your arms, lower your body until your elbows are at 90 degrees. Push back up. Keep your head and chin up during the process.

Crab Walk

- o Get down into a crab position: hands and feet in line with each other and flat on the ground with your chest facing up not down, knees bent, and hips held several inches off the ground. Walk several spaces forward, and then several spaces back.

Narrow-width Pushups

- ○ Narrowing your hand placement while completing pushups will engage your core while toning your triceps, pectorals, and shoulders. Start in a pushup position, but instead of your hands lining up with your shoulders, move them in slightly on both sides. Lower your body down, holding yourself up, then push back into the starting position.

Focus: Legs

Wall Sit

- ○ Set your back up against a stable wall until your knees form a 90-degree angle with the wall. Your head, shoulders, and upper back should be lying flat against the wall, with your weight evenly distributed between both feet.

Jump Squat

- ○ Standing straight up, keep your arms down by your sides. Squat down normally until your upper thighs are as close to parallel with the floor as they can be. Pressing off with your feet, jump straight up into the air, and as you touch down, go back into the squatting position and start again.

Lunges

- ○ Starting in a standing position, head and chin up, eyes forward, take a step forward with one leg ensuring your knee is above your ankle. You don't want your other knee to touch the ground. Push back up into standing position and step forward with your opposite leg.

Focus: Chest

Incline Pushups

- o   This form is a great modification for those who may just be beginning and are struggling to do a basic pushup. Find some kind of incline in your workout area: a desk, wall, chair, etc. and stand facing the incline with your feet shoulder width apart and feet 1-2 feet back from the wall. Place your hands on either side of the incline and place them slightly wider than your shoulders. Slowly bend the elbows and lower your body toward the incline, pause and push back up—try not to lock your elbows.

Traditional Plank

- o   Start off in a pushup position. Instead of lowering yourself and pushing yourself back up, you intend to hold your body in that position. Do not bend your elbows and make sure your feet are not wider than your shoulders. Hold this pose for 10 seconds to begin, and as you begin to master this exercise, work your way up to 30 seconds, 1 minute, etc.

Burpees

- o   This move combines several moves into one and can be a killer workout for beginners. Standing straight up, bend down in a position with your hands on the floor supporting your body. Kick back both feet until you are in a plank/pushup position.

Quickly jump back on your feet and spring up, raising your hands to the sky. After lowering your arms, start again by bending back down.

Focus: Back

Reverse Snow Angel

○ Instead of lying on your back like you were about to make a snow angel, flip over and lay face down on the ground. Raise your arms and shoulders off the ground slightly, about two inches, and bring your hands down from your sides up past your head. (If you were standing not laying down you would be raising and lowering your arms in an up and down wing-flapping motion.)

Superman

○ Lie face down on the ground with your toes pointing down under your body. Reach your arms out straight to your sides, and raise both your arms and feet in the air while making sure your torso maintains contact with the ground.

Good Mornings aka Hip Hinges

○ Standing up straight with your hands on your hips and your feet shoulder-width apart, bend forward at your waist until your back is parallel to the ground. Engage your core and bring your torso back up in a straight position. It is important to keep your neck in line with your spine while doing this exercise.

Focus: Butt

Fire Hydrants

○ Start in a modified pushup position—the standard pushup position but with knees and hands on the ground instead of feet and hands on the ground. Raise one leg off the ground with your knee bent at a 90-degree angle. This move can also be completed with a straight leg for similar results. If you need inspiration, you want to look like a dog who is just about the use a fire hydrant!

Leg Kickbacks

○ Again, start in a modified pushup position. Try to align your shoulders with your knees. Kick one leg back behind you. Make sure you feel the movement in your hips and glutes, not your lower back. Bring your leg back down and switch sides.

Glute Bridges

○ Lay on the ground, flat on your back with your hands by your sides. Place your feet flat on the floor shoulder-width apart. Use your upper back, upper arms, and core to raise your hips up off the ground toward the sky while keeping your feet and arms on the ground. Slowly lower your hips until they are resting back on the ground.

Focus: Abs

Side Planks

- o Lie down on your side on the floor, and place one elbow underneath you so that you are forming a plank on one side. Keeping your elbow underneath your shoulder, push your lower torso up off of the ground so that the only things touching the ground are your right forearm and the side of your right foot or your left forearm and the side of your left foot. Hold the position for ten seconds, release, and then resume the position.

Flutter Kicks

- o Lie on your back on the floor with your arms down by your sides and your heels flat on the ground. Lift your heels about 6 inches off the ground, and quickly kick your legs up and down. It is easier to complete 10 kicks, rest for 20 seconds, then do another 10 kicks because of how short and quick the kicks are.

V-Sit Crunch

- o Lay flat on your back on the ground with your arms laying above your head. Lift up your legs like you are about to attempt a crunch, but bring your arms up toward your legs at the same time, creating a 'V.' Lower your arms and legs back into the starting position lying down.

Summary and Key Points

There are many more exercises within each focus category. The ones listed in this book are just suggestions to get you started.

If you are confused about how to complete an exercise, YouTube has an excellent variety of step-by-step videos.

It's a great idea to track your repetitions (reps), so you know you started being able to do 10 pushups and now doing 25!

Chapter 3: Planning a Workout Routine That Works For You

Bodyweight workouts are perfect because it can be completed with only some space and your body: no gym or equipment required! An even better bonus to these exercises is that they are so simple to do that they are easily combined to reap even more benefits in the same amount of time.

What to Include In Your Plan

Important aspects of a workout routine include duration, frequency, intensity, and consistency. The Mayo Clinic suggests adults get in about 150 minutes of moderate exercise a week, or 75 minutes of vigorous activity and at least 2 days of strength training: "Moderate aerobic exercise includes activities such as brisk walking, swimming, and mowing the lawn. Vigorous aerobic exercise includes activities such as running and aerobic dancing. Strength training can include the use of weight machines, your own body weight, resistance tubing, resistance paddles in the water, or activities such as rock climbing."

To break this down for you, you should look at workouts with moderate intensity for 3 days a week for 50 minutes each, or 5 days a week for 30 minutes each. It's up to you to decide when you want to schedule your workouts throughout the week, but making sure you start your Mondays with a workout is always a great way to set up your week for success!

How to Stay Dedicated When Your Resolve Falters

A LifeHacker article written by Alan Henry has some great tips on how to motivate yourself to start your routine and how to stick with your routine. Without consistency, you will never see or keep results!

1. Stop Making Excuses

    Don't be too hard on yourself, we all make mistakes and expect too much from ourselves. Know that failures are an expected part of the journey.

    We all have to start from somewhere—doing something, no matter how small, is better than doing nothing at all!

2. Understand Your Habits

    "Most people fail in fitness because they never enter a self-sustaining positive feedback loop. To be successful at fitness, it needs to be in the same category of the brain as sleeping, eating, and sex." The key is to find a routine replacement that works for you and gets results for the energy you put into building it into your habits."

    Starting from zero can cause people to want to give up: "Oftentimes, people are actually lazy because they're out of shape and don't exercise!" It's quite easy for a fit person to tell someone who's having a tough time that they're just lazy, but the reality is that running a mile is much easier for someone who does five every day compared to someone who's been sitting on the couch for most of his life."

3. Find Your "Secret Sauce"

"Minimizing and oversimplifying the challenge doesn't help, and while hearing what worked for others can help you figure out things to try, it's almost never going to be exactly what works for you. Look for your own combination of tools, tips, techniques, and advice that will support you and your health and fitness goals."

4. Be Engaged and Stick to Your Plan

"Set the bar low and start small. If you're having trouble with working out every day, start with twice or once a week. Whatever it is, start with something you can *definitely* do effortlessly. This is where suggestions like parking on the far end of the lot and taking the stairs come into play."

"Whatever you do, make it fun. Whatever you do, enjoy it. Choose something rewarding enough to make you feel good about doing it. If you're having a good time, mistakes feel like learning experiences and challenges to be overcome, not throw-up-your-hands-and-give-up moments."

5. Track Your Victories With Technology

"Technology can be a huge benefit to help you see your progress in a way that looking in the mirror won't show you. The goal is to keep that track record, whether it's on a calendar, in an app, or on a website, going unbroken as long as possible. Just remember, quantifying your efforts is just a method to get feedback and track your progress. Your tech should be a means to build better habits, not the habit in itself."

Another great way to keep yourself accountable is by enlisting a friend to work out with you. Even if you don't have the same fitness goals or you don't want to be distracted while you are trying to work out, having someone to be accountable to can really push us to meet our goals. Whether that's a text or a phone call on days you know your friend should be working out, that small reminder may be enough to get them going.

Sample 7-day Routine

After deciding how many days and for how long each day you want to work out, the next step is planning what exercises you will complete in each session. It's not generally recommended that you focus on the same muscle groups two days in a row, although every other day is absolutely fine!

Sunday: Arms

  15 pushups x3

  15 tricep dips x3

  15 lay down pushup x3

  15 walkouts x3

Monday: Legs

  15 jump squats x3

  16 X jumps x3

  15 lunges x3

  24 high knees x3

10 burpees x3

Tuesday: Rest!

Wednesday: Chest

10 second plank x3

15 decline pushups x3

15 mountain climbers x3

15 burpees x3

Thursday: Abs

15 straight leg sit ups x3

20 ab bikes x3

15 straight leg raises x3

20 side twists

Friday: Rest!

Saturday: Back

15 bridges x3

15 back extensions x3

15 opposite arm/leg raises x3

15 bridges x3

Try to complete all four workouts on each day as fast as you can while resting for up to 30 seconds between each move. If you want to up the intensity, slowly increase the repetitions—a good interval is an increase of 5. Another way to make the workout more intense is to complete the workout as a circuit. If you complete a day's workouts as a circuit, ignore the "repeat 3 times." Instead, you would complete, for example, 15 straight leg sit-ups, 20 ab bikes, 15 straight leg raises, and 20 side twists. Rest for 30 seconds! Repeat starting with 15 straight leg sit-ups. Try to not rest for more than 30 seconds. If you need to when you're just beginning, that's completely okay! Complete one circuit and begin working on adding additional circuits to your workouts.

If you already have a workout routine that you regularly complete, try adding in certain strength training exercises between your cardio workout. Again, slowly build up your repetitions but starting small.

Summary and Key Points

> Plan your workouts into your day with your planner or calendar system. Start small and build your way up to working out 3, 4, or 5 days a week!

> Switch up the muscle groups you focus on to make sure that you see full body results.

> The recommended workouts are only a very small example of workouts within each category to get you started. Research muscle groups you want to target and incorporate those goals into your workout plan.

Chapter 4: How to Make the Most Out of Your Bodyweight Workouts

As touched on in the last chapter regarding circuit workouts, High-Intensity Interval Training is a great way to target multiple muscle groups in one workout and burn more calories. We will also touch on tools that can be used to track your workouts and your progress, as well as an important aspect of ending your workout that is sometimes forgotten but still important: stretching!

High-Intensity Interval Training

According to Bodybuilding.com, "these different body compositions point to the fact that not all cardio is created equal, which is why it's important to choose a form of cardio that meets your goals. A recent study compared participants who did steady-state cardio for 30 minutes three times a week to those who did 20 minutes of high-intensity interval training (HIIT) three times per week. Both groups showed similar weight loss, but the HIIT group showed a 2 percent loss in body fat while the steady-state group lost only 0.3 percent. The HIIT group also gained nearly two pounds of muscle, while the steady-state group lost almost a pound."

Photo by Autumn Goodman on Unsplash

Progress Can Be Small, But Any Progress is Significant

Tracking your gains is an important part of using body weight workouts. Some people prefer creating their own systems in a notebook or journal, others use electronic devices, and the rest of us prefer to use visual progress indicators.

Writing down when you completed a workout, what exercises you completed, and how many repetitions you completed is a great reminder of your goals and how far you've come on the journey to reach them. Before your next workout, refer back to your last logged workout and see what adjustments you need to make to your workout today to help you be successful.

Technology Can Help Us Keep More Accurate Records

Using a tracking device like a Fitbit watch, hybrid smartwatch, iPhone, or smart shoes, you can track calories burned, distance moved, heart rate, and then have them saved somewhere digitally instead of in a hard copy paper form.

Stretching for Injury Prevention Should Be a Priority

Warming up and then stretching after a workout is an important way to help prevent injuries. Stretch out your arms, legs, back, and any other areas that feel tight.

Key Summary Points

HIIT workouts are a great way to combine targeting different muscle groups in one workout instead of many.

Tracking your gains in whichever fashion makes you the most comfortable and that you find the most motivating is highly encouraged!

Taking 5-15 minutes to stretch after a workout will ease soreness for your workouts in the following days, and will help prevent your muscles from getting injured.

PART 2

Chapter One: Muscle Mass

You have probably heard by now of the many benefits of having more of your body being composed of muscle mass. And yet, I'd venture to guess you still don't know the half of it!

If you're a woman, thirty percent of your body is made up of muscle mass; for men, it's around forty. The bottom line is, we all want more muscle! Muscle gives us that long and lean appearance—with nicely shaped muscles. Muscular people are viewed as healthy people. Obviously, they are also stronger. Too much fat can lead to all kinds of health problems, not to mention all the clothes you have that you can't wear!

There are many, many reasons to desire to build more muscle, but I'll give you the one that is at the top of the list for me: muscle burns fat. That's right! Muscle burns fat not only when you're in the gym or somewhere else, hitting the weights, or doing body resistance training, it does so when you're at rest. That is correct. Muscle eats away at fat while you're lolling on the sofa watching that Sunday afternoon football game.

This is why we love muscle!

Many folks don't do weight training because they think they have to head to the gym. It's a very common myth that it's necessary to use weights in order to add muscle. But it's just that—a myth. You also don't have to purchase a room full of expensive weights, gadgets and other equipment to use to build muscle at home.

I'm going to let you in on a little secret. You can build muscle using just...you. It is true. You can use your own body's resistance against itself to burn fat and build muscle. It's awesome! This way, there are no excuses. You don't have to pay a gym membership, drive yourself there, or even leave the comfort of your own home.

I'm going to give you nine different muscle-building, fat-burning workouts, and we're going to talk—just a little—about a few things you can do in the area of diet. Yes, diet. Not "diet" as in a bad word—like "I feel miserable after eating badly for the last two weeks and I need to go on a diet." Not that sort of talk. We'll simply touch on some of the foods you should be eating and some of the food you shouldn't be if you're genuinely interested in losing some weight.

Before we get into the exercises, let's cover some basics.

How Muscle is Built

Simply put in laymen's terms, when you work out, you essentially damage your muscles. Muscle tissue is broken down. When this process happens, your body gets busy repairing and replacing these damaged tissues. To get just a little technical during this process, the body has a process on the cellular level in which it repairs or replaces the damaged muscle fibers. It fuses these fibers together to form new myofibrils (muscle protein strands). Repaired myofibrils are larger in thickness and are greater in number, thus causing muscle hypertrophy (growth). This process doesn't happen when you are lifting weights, though. It happens afterward when the body is at rest. That's why rest is absolutely a key component to muscle growth.

The hard work is only half the process. But fortunately the rest—pun intended—is easy.

Chapter Two: The Upper Body

"Can we please have a moment of silence for all those stuck in traffic on the way to the gym?" —Anonymous

These aren't always the easiest exercises to do—well, actually, exercising isn't exactly easy anyway, so scratch that. The great thing about upper body work is that this is where you will begin to see results first. So, for that reason, doing upper body work can be incredibly rewarding.

1. The Classic Push-Up

Push-ups are super easy, super basic and have been around forever. The reason they've been around forever is that they're also super effective. The key is to perform them correctly. If you don't, they become wasted effort.

The proper way to do push-ups

Get on the ground, belly down. Place your palms on the floor a shoulder width apart or slightly more. Keep your body straight as you push yourself up by extending your arms. Repeat. Make sure that your arms are lifting your body weight, not the muscles on the lower half of your body. Imagine there is a plank of wood on your back starting from your head to your feet. Make sure that your body is as straight as that plank in order to maintain correct body alignment.

How many push-ups?

That depends on the kind of shape you are in when you start. When you begin to do the push-ups, do they feel easy to you? Make sure you are performing the move deliberately—not going too fast that you're using momentum. The first time you try, do as many as you can while still keeping perfect form. Afterward, for your regular sets, do two-thirds that many. So, if you did fifteen but were tired by then and beginning to lose form, use ten as a target for your sets in the beginning.

As you get stronger, make the number higher. You want to continue to be challenged. Some people do as many as one-hundred push-ups per day. Perhaps that's something you can aim for. For the average beginner, three sets of ten are reasonable.

2. Chair-Dips

This is another upper-body exercise that, while in actuality, you're using your body-weight, you'll still need a chair or a bench or something similar. When I'm out running, there's a square cement planter that has an edge to it, and it works perfectly.

Dips further work the rhomboid muscles in your back and synchronize with push-ups on working your triceps.

Get a chair/bench or another object capable of supporting your body weight and of a similar height, as explained above. Stand with your back to it. Make sure that the object is sturdy enough to support your entire body weight. Lower yourself and place your palms on the front edge of the bench, fingers pointing forward. Tuck in your elbows to your sides. Maintain this position and walk just your feet slowly in front of you. Your body weight should be resting on your arms now. Deliberately bend your arms and lower yourself. Do this until the floor is parallel to your upper arms. If you're doing it right, you'll feel it in your back and also in your triceps. Simply hold for about a second and return to the starting position.

Do three sets. Determine the number of repetitions per set the exact same way as you did for the push-ups.

3. Diamond Push-Ups

Oh, chicken wings—and not the kind you eat. "Chicken wing" is a common term used to refer to the fat on the back of a person's upper arm as it kind of tends to sag, resulting in an unattractive "flapping in the wind" sort of scenario when you wave your arms. Nobody has time for this, people! Not when there are exercises that will blast those wings if you simply stay consistent. Almost everyone wants tight, toned arms. It's a sexy look, and it's youthful! Tight triceps can actually defy a woman's age. So don't skimp on the upper body exercises. I'm giving you three here, and all of them work your triceps, but the Diamond Push-Up works it the most of all so if you're only worried about triceps and nothing else, do this one.

Start in the push-up position, yet instead of having your hands out to the sides, place them in front of you and put them together to create a diamond shape.

Raise yourself until your legs are straight then lower yourself until you are two inches above the ground. You will feel the burn in those triceps. Embrace the burn! The burn means the move is working.

Choose your number of reps in the same manner with all of the upper body exercises.

Chapter Three: The Core

You must not ignore the importance of core work when it comes to resistance training. Your core muscles are the ones that essentially holds everything else together.

There's a very good chance that, no matter what you're doing, you're using your core. Having a weak core takes the power away from all the rest of your muscles. Your core muscles are also responsible for your balance and stability, which is huge. Your core is not one muscle; it's a complicated interconnected series of muscles which effectively include all of them except your arms and your legs. So, I reiterate. Working your core needs to be an incredibly important part of your exercise routine.

Think about your abs. Everybody seems to be concerned with their abdominal muscles. Many people want those six-pack muscles to show. Some just want to button their favorite jeans without lying on the bed.

There's a common misconception (still) that fat can be "spot-burned." This is simply not true. The general consensus is that fat leaves the body the same way it came on—gradually and kind of all over. Don't get me wrong on this; genetics do play a role in how our bodies store fat. Some people can be perfectly proportioned pretty much everywhere on their bodies and yet have large, unattractive bellies. Those people are still more the exception than the rule.

So, the bottom line is that you cannot target fat-burning. If you really want the fat to leave your body, there are three central areas that will require your attention: diet, cardio, and resistance training. Here we are focusing on the third, and a little later I'm going to give a quick overall snapshot of the importance of combining all three.

I'm going to give you three exercises for your core. This first one, known as a Plank, could actually be used as the only core exercise you do. It is that effective and, especially considering the other exercises you'll be doing with, will touch all the muscles in your core.

Now, remember what we said about abs and fat? Here's something many people simply don't realize. Underneath however much fat we happen to be carrying on our abdominal muscles, we all have a "six-pack." Those are muscles in each of our bodies. What people are trying to do when they say they're going for six-pack abs is burn the layers of fat that cover those muscles. As I said, and much to the sadness of myself and many others, you can't target that weight.

Additionally, I'm not going to include any kind of "sit-ups" in upper body work. They've been proven to not be as effective as other exercises that work the core muscles. Also, I personally think that unless your form is always perfect with a sit-up, you may be putting certain back muscles at risk.

4. Plank

This one is tough, but like I said, with this one exercise and all the many variations you can do with it, you can get those core muscles strong in no time.

Start with the initial push-up position. Bend your elbows to a right angle. Let your weight rest on your forearms. You might want to get a mat or something soft to use as padding between your arms and the floor. Make sure you have a timer too. The elbows need to be beneath your shoulders directly. Your body should be forming a straight line from head to heels—like a plank. Hold this position for as long as you can without injuring yourself.

Your goal should eventually be to hold it for two minutes. I said eventually for a good reason. Planks are tough. I mean, for a lot of people, a ten-second plank and they're toast. Because so many muscles are used to hold this position, if those muscles aren't strong, it simply can't happen for very long. That's also why planks are such a good indicator of how far you've come. If, when you start it takes all you have to hold a thirty-second plank, I would venture to guess that after a religiously followed routine, within eight weeks you will have worked up to the full two minutes.

Planks are great because there are many variations of them, as well. As you get stronger, try this:

While in plank position, lift one of your legs as high as you can and hold it there for a count of thirty. Repeat on the other side.

You can even do a side plank. Lay down on your side with your head propped on your elbow, raise your body in that position and hold it. To increase difficulty with this one, once you are in the up position, try raising your top leg and holding it in that position.

Planks can be thought of as a "Super Move." They literally work all of your muscles. In fact, if one really wanted to, one could do planks only as their resistance training (planks in all their variations, which are many) and achieve the results they're looking for.

5. *Reverse Crunch*

Okay, so I realize I just got done telling you that sit-ups, which are essentially crunches, are not good for the back muscles. In fact, one physician has said that he has seen no other cause of back injury with the highest rate as traditional crunches.

However, the reverse crunch, despite its name, does not carry the same risks and is excellent at targeting your abdominal muscles.

Here's how to do it:

> Lie down on the floor and fully extend your arms and legs to the sides. Put your palms on the floor. Your arms should actually stay in one place as you perform the entire exercise.

> This is the position you will start from: your legs will be pulled up which will make your thighs form a right angle with the floor. You will want your feet together and also parallel to the floor.

> Move your legs towards your torso. At the same time, roll your pelvis backward. Raise your hips above the floor. The goal is to have your knees touching your chest.

> Hold this position for around a second, then lower back to the starting position.

Again, depending on your ability when you start, gauge the number of reps and sets by how they feel to your body and how hard it is for you to do them at first. Just make sure not to overestimate yourself too much. Muscle soreness from overdoing it is no fun!

6. *Mountain Climber*

Get into the top of the push-up position. This is the starting position.

Keeping your back in a straight line, bring your right knee toward your chest. Quickly bring it back to the starting position. Do the same for the left knee. Repeat but speed up the movement, alternating legs quickly as if you were running in place with your hands on the ground.

As far as how many sets, this move isn't exactly structured that way so use seconds to guide you. Try the move until you are really struggling to continue (you'll likely be out of breath) then use two-thirds of those seconds, call it a set, and do three.

Chapter Four: The Lower Body

Working out your lower body is not to be taken lightly or skimped on when doing resistance training. One particular reason for this is because your lower body contains the largest muscle in your entire body: the gluteus maximus.

Not only do most of us like to work out this muscle because it makes us "look" better, it's also a powerhouse. This muscle, along with other gluteal muscles, is one of the great stabilizers of the human body. Keeping these muscles strong can minimize aches and pains in your lower back and hips. The muscles also give you the power you need to do simple things like walk, run, and climb.

So, whenever lower body resistance training is discussed, there are two moves that are practically givens. No, it's not because they're both somewhat torturous—it's because they are effective!

When you're doing your workout, never forget the old adage, "Pain is temporary…(fill in the blank)." Usually, people say, "pain is temporary, quitting lasts forever."

That doesn't exactly apply here, but the point is that if you aren't going to be able to tolerate a little bit of pain, you aren't going to get the same results. Workouts can hurt. Muscles burn. Sometimes by the end of a good workout, you feel like you're about to croak. As far as I'm concerned, those are the very best kind! It means you've really kicked some gluteal maximuses and made some progress for the day. You have to maintain a good attitude if you're going to embark on this journey.

Results don't happen overnight, but relatively you will start to see them very quickly (although, in general people who are close to you will notice before you do.) However, nothing is more satisfying than when you do look in the mirror and see results that can't be denied, or when you put on a pair of jeans that has been an eternity since they were last wore and they button easily. It's a powerful feeling.

So, here they come, the not-always-fun but ever-so-productive lower body movements.

7. The Lunge

If you've ever done them, you're probably feeling the burn simply at the thought! When executed correctly, these babies do burn, but they are incredibly effective.

Lunges produce fast results. You will notice that your legs and derriere are more toned and attractive looking. You will feel that you're stronger and you'll notice the difference when you do cardio—assuming you do, of course.

Lunges do not require weights, although weights can be added later on to increase the difficulty as you get into better shape.

Form in lunges is very important. The same is true with all of these exercises. If you're going to put in the effort, you may as well make sure you're doing it right in order to maximize your results.

Following is how to execute a perfect lunge:

> Stand upright and keep your body straight. Pull your shoulders back and relax your chin. Keep your chin pointed forward, don't look down. Make sure the muscles in your core are tight and engaged.

If it helps you with balance, you can use something you have on hand, like, say, a broom. Hold it crossways in front of you and let it lightly rest on your shoulders.

Pick a leg. Step forward using that leg. Lower your hips until both your knees are forming a right angle. Make sure that your lowered knee isn't touching the floor and that your forward knee is directly above your angle and not too far forward. Make sure that your weight is in your heels as you push yourself back up to the starting position.

When you do push back up to the starting position, really place extra emphasis on engaging your gluteus maximus. Deliberately use the strength in that muscle to push yourself upright.

Now. Repeat. How many times? I recommend starting with three sets of ten perfectly executed lunges. If you don't feel "the burn" add a couple, or go ahead and use a barbell if you have one and put some weight on it. You can even do lunges in reverse, to vary things up.

8. Squat

Ah, the squat. If you haven't done them, you've probably heard of them if you have any friends at all who work out. Like lunges, they are simple, easy to execute, and incredibly effective at increasing muscle mask and making you stronger.

Also, like lunges, there are quite a few variations to squats that you can use as you get more fit. For now, of course, we'll focus on the simple squat. Again, form is super important.

Stand with your feet at least shoulder-width apart. If you feel more comfortable, it's okay to place your feet a bit wider apart. As you stand, you should focus on having your weight on your heels. Extend your arms straight out. The first thing you'll do is thrust your hips back slightly as though you are about to take a seat. Then, lower yourself down like that as if you are actually about to sit down. You'll want to go as low as you can. The goal is to make your knees bent so that your legs are parallel to the floor, again almost if you were sitting in a chair. Control your knees so they don't move forward over your feet.

The next step is simply to stand up, and when you are coming upright, squeeze your glutes at the top of the movement. So, essentially, squats are like sitting in an invisible chair, then standing up using your glutes to propel you. Very easy but super effective!

9. The Bridge

The bridge is another great one for strengthening your glutes and legs. Remember, before you even see the results of these exercises, you'll be stronger for doing them. And, if you eat right and take in enough protein (building blocks for muscle) you will increase the size of your muscle and consequently burn fat. So when you're doing these not-so-fun-at-the-time moves, keep that in mind!

Here's how to do a bridge: Lie on the floor, flat as a pancake. Place your hands on your sides and bend your knees. Your feet should be about shoulder-width apart. Lift your hips off the floor, using your heels to push. Keep your back straight while doing this! Hold the position for a second and squeeze those glutes.

Slowly lower back to the position you started from.

For the number of reps, use the method we discussed previously. The first time you try the exercise, go until you really feel the burn—until it's very tough to continue or until you would not be able to. However many reps that is (say it's fifteen) subtract one-third of that number and start from there.

For variety, this exercise can be performed with one leg at a time.

Chapter Five: Putting it all Together

People have different preferences in how they like to work out. To see good results from strength training, you need to work each muscle group no less than two times per week. Three times is fine and you may see faster results that way. Depending on what you want to accomplish, generally, three times is enough.

The idea is to give each muscle group a rest day in between your workouts. So people go about the entire construct differently. Some like to work their entire body in one session, then rest for a day or two and do it again, up to three times a week.

Others prefer to break the muscle group workouts up. Legs one day, arms the next, core the next, like that.

In my opinion and in consideration of the research I've done, any of the above-mentioned ways to go about it will be just as effective as another. Of course, the most important component is that it gets done.

I'd like to take a moment at the time to talk about cardiovascular workouts. I know, I know, boo, hiss. A lot of people really aren't that big on cardio. However, there's a lot to be said for a good cardio sweat session. For one thing, cardiovascular exercise improves the health of our heart and lungs. That alone should be reason enough to work some in. Also, this type of exercise, depending on the type you choose, can burn an awful lot of calories. Remember, any calories burned will contribute to that sleek, muscular look. For the muscles to come out, the fat has to come off.

Cardiovascular exercise has also been proven to affect our moods in a positive way (the same can be said for weight training.)

The best, most well-rounded exercise plans include a mixture of both. Supposing you hate cardio, you will do yourself no harm by keeping it to a minimum. The general recommendation right now is to get thirty minutes of cardio on "most" days of the week.

Given that, as an example, you could do your weights on Monday, cardio Tuesday, weights Wednesday, Cardio Thursday, weights Friday and guess what? Take the weekend off!

This is just one example of how this can all be done. You can be as creative as you want to be or as you need to be to get around a work schedule.

You could do, for instance, cardio in the morning and resistance training at night. You could work in all or part of your resistance training during your lunch hour at work.

There are no limits to the options available, so that simply means *no excuses*.

No equipment or anything fancy is required for the cardio portion either. Walking is cardio. Just walk fast enough to get your heart rate up, break a sweat and breathe a little heavy. Increase intensity as your fitness level improves.

Here's a sample plan, if you need one. I'm going to use ten reps as a standard while performing the strength training for the sake of simplicity.

Monday Morning Before Work:

Three sets of ten of each of the following:

Push-ups

Chair-Dips

Diamond Push-ups

Honestly, this should take you no more than ten minutes.

Monday Lunch:

Walk for thirty minutes

Monday Evening:

Perform three sets of the following:

Squats

Lunges

Bridges

Planks

Mountain Climber

Reverse Crunch

Starting out, repeat this same routine on Wednesdays and Fridays. Try this for a few weeks (or another plan of your own design) and see how it works with your schedule.

On the days that you don't walk for thirty-minutes on your lunch, per your official "schedule," do it anyway. If not that, jump on the trampoline with your little ones at night for half an hour. Ride your bike. Swim. Ski if you live near snow and/or if it's wintertime. Snow Show. Or...head to the gym. Do the elliptical or the stair-climber for half of an hour. It's really not hard to get in the minimum amount of cardio and depending on your goals, and who says you have to stop with the minimum?

If you stick to this program, you're going to see some results and you'll see them pretty quickly.

Here's another tip: throw away your scale. Okay, well you don't have to throw it away. I just don't recommend weighing yourself all the time. It could discourage you in fact, for the simple reason that muscle actually does weigh more than fat. You might gain in the beginning, and no one wants to start a workout program only to see the numbers on the scale go up. No way! Instead of worrying about the scale, judge your progress by—most importantly—how you feel, and as for changes in your body, you can always take some initial measurements and then re-measure once a week. What has always worked best for me is simply to gauge how my clothes fit. That's the biggest tell of all. I have a pair of jean shorts I'm wearing right now. A couple of months ago I couldn't get them to even think about zipping! That's the only kind of progress I need. To me, numbers on the scale don't mean a whole lot.

Chapter Six: On Your Diet

It wouldn't be right to talk about gaining muscle and losing fat without talking a bit about diet.

I'm not going to go overboard but there are a few things I'd like to touch on.

First off, as I previously spoke about at the end of chapter four—the scale—I forgot to mention another reason I don't care to use them. Most of them have a tendency to fluctuate as much as five pounds in less than twenty-four hours. In other words, if I'm going by the scale, I often will have "gained" five pounds from when I got up to when it's time for bed.

Not cool.

Not possible, either. Our bodies are made up of an estimated sixty-five percent water. It is normal for the amount of water in our bodies to fluctuate all the time.

Losing water weight does not equate to losing fat. However, while we are trying to lose weight, and while we're working out, it is especially important to keep our bodies hydrated.

There are as many theories on the web as you could click on about how much water to drink, but for questions like these, I like to refer to the Mayo Clinic website, because I know that the information they put out here has been thoroughly researched. What follows is their advice on water intake:

48

Every single day, you lose water by breathing, sweating, urinating, and pooping. To
function properly, your body's water must be replenished through the consumption of food and beverages.

The average healthy man who lives in a temperate climate needs 15.5 cups or 3.7
liters of fluids every day, and the average healthy woman living in the same place needs 11.5 cups or 2.7 liters every day.

This is about what I do for myself in a normal day and it seems to work.
Regardless, don't skimp on the water.

There's another important factor when it comes to building muscle and that's protein. If you are serious about adding some muscle mass, you're going to need to eat your protein. That doesn't mean it has to be meat; there are plenty of non-meat options for protein intake. Of course, if you are a vegetarian you already know that.

Another little tip: your body needs fat to lose fat. Sounds strange, doesn't it? But if your body is starved of nutrients, it will begin to hold on to everything it has instinctually, and as a result, you won't see any weight loss.

There are a million types of "diets" out there, and this is not a book about diets so
I'm not going to delve into them. If I were going to say anything at all about your
diet (and don't get me wrong, your diet IS important,) I would say two words: eat clean.

What does that mean? Since clean is the opposite of dirty, in this case, think dirty equals "processed."

49

Do your body a giant favor and stay away from processed foods! Eat foods that are as "close" to the earth as you can.

Lean proteins (including fish and non-meat proteins)

Tons—and I do really mean tons—of vegetables

Lean fat (avocado, almonds, coconut oi

l) Dairy (full-fat; eat sparingly)

Fruits (sparingly)

It's that simple. No "TV Dinners." No boxes of macaroni and cheese, ple ase.
Nothing that has a "bunch" of ingredients, many of which you aren't even fa miliar with. Those are bad. Leave them in the store.

If you have a sweet tooth, indulge it, but rarely, and even a sweet tooth c an be
indulged in a healthy manner. There's nothing wrong with eating some strawberri es topped with full fat whipped cream. Yummy!

Well, there you have it. You really are set. Everything is explained and con densed for you.

Start your weight training and your cardio, eat clean, drink your water and r eap the rewards.

Go   get   'em!

50

PART 3

Chapter 1: How to Choose the Right Number of Repetitions

"How do I choose the number of repetitions and series?"

This is one of the main doubts that assail the neophytes of the gym. I still remember the day I asked my gym instructor about it many years ago. In fact, the first questions that a beginner poses to the instructor in front of a weight machine are typically these: "How many consecutive lifts (or movements) do I have to do with this machines? And for how many times?"

The most precise ones even dare to ask how much time they have to recover from one set to the next one, and so you think you have clarified everything you need to know about a training session at a given weight machine.

The load (i.e., the kg lifted or moved) is generally fixed according to the presumed abilities of the aspiring visitor of the weight room, often without any relation to the first two parameters of repetitions and sets.

There is not a unique answer to these questions since it all depends on the goal. For example, when I first started my training journey, I wanted to get bigger, not stronger. During that period I did a lot of hypertrophy-oriented workouts which worked quite well. When I switched to a more strength-oriented approach, I had to completely rearrange my schedule all over again.

Since the weight training that interests us is not aimed at the practice of bodybuilding—but is framed in the health of those who want to integrate aerobic activities with exercises for the general improvement of strength, elasticity, and flexibility—before defining the number of repetitions and sets, it is necessary to establish the objective to be achieved or what aspect do you want to train for between the following:

The resistant force: the force that the muscle must apply to overcome the fatigue resulting from a prolonged effort.

The maximal force: the maximum force that the muscle can develop with a lifting test (or a limited number of tests). It is also often referred to as a maximal load if referring to a specific exercise in the gym.

The fast force: the maximum force that the muscle can develop to counteract a load in a limited period of time. Referring to time, therefore, more than force we should speak of power which is the ability to develop a force in the unity of time.

Muscle hypertrophy: no reference is made to the type of force that the muscle has to generate, but to its effect on the athlete's body—that is, to maximize the increase in muscle volume. The muscular volume is connected to the developed force, because the greater the cross section of the muscle, the greater the muscle fibers available to make the effort. However, the equation *muscle hypertrophy = greater muscle strength* is not always true because, in addition to having available muscle fibers, the human body must also know how to recruit, and this is influenced by other factors such as the efficiency of the cardio-respiratory system, the ability coordination, etc. This should make those who seek to maximize muscle hypertrophy think only of achieving the highest possible performance.

In a healthy view of strength training, you can leave out the last point because the search for muscle hypertrophy, typical of bodybuilders, is far from our goals. Therefore, we can identify three types of training, each of which corresponds to a type of strength that you want to train and, consequently, to a pattern of repetitions-number of sets-interval between the different series.

Remember that to define a training plan, the following variables must be defined for each exercise (i.e., for each machine in the gym or exercise with weights):

Repetition: it is the single gesture of weightlifting or athletic gesture that stresses the muscle or a district of the muscles. Generally, in the gym at each repetition, the muscle or muscles lift or move a weight (load).

Sets: the consecutive number of repetitions. The set can be slow or fast, or the exercise is done slowly, calmly, or quickly, imposing to adhere to a higher rhythm.

Recovery: the time between one series and the next.

So, you might find a typical 3-row workout of 12 sets of 25 kg with a three-minute recovery. This is a very standard way to get started and the first style of training that I followed when started out.

Chapter 2: How to Breathe During Exercises

One thing that is often overlooked by many gym enthusiasts is how to perform proper breathing during weight exercises. It is a problem that, sooner or later, most of those who attend gyms propose to their instructor.

Breathing, as we know, is an activity that we do involuntarily, but it is also possible to control it trying to adapt the movement of the muscles (or part of the muscles) involved, such as the diaphragm, the ribcage, the shoulders, abdominals to the rhythm that we want to follow.

Consciously, one can control the inhalation phase and the exhalation phase in their overall duration or even suspend breathing by entering apnoea.

A lot of sports and disciplines (yoga, pilates, etc.), give a lot of importance to breathing, while other oriental disciplines even give it a spiritual value.

Even in the exercises that are performed in the gym, including those with weights, breathing has a considerable importance. Unfortunately, there are not many who have clear ideas about it.

Instructors usually advise to:

inhale in the discharge phase of the action, usually when the weight is being returned to its initial position;

exhale in the loading phase of the exercise or when there is more effort required.

This usually works well, even if the beginner will at first see this as another constraint which will only confuse him. In reality, it requires a good amount of concentration to force yourself to control breathing in this way and therefore forces the athlete to give complete attention to what he is doing. A lot of times, people look around in the gym while doing an exercise, or—worse—talking to someone. This is something that I have never understood: to me, strength training is a way to become the best version of myself, both physically and mentally, and I do not have time to waste. Focusing on breathing is a good way to think exclusively about the exercise you are performing.

The following is a good general rule to follow:

The most important thing to do is not to hold your breath during the loading phase.

Holding your breath in the loading phase is a big mistake, as it is instinctive to hold your breath during the maximum effort required. Instead, the opposite must be done because this practice can also lead to serious consequences, especially if the effort involves muscles of the upper body.

Holding the breath deliberately blocks the glottis, which then leads to a compression of the veins due to an increase in pressure inside the ribcage. As a result of this compression, the veins can also partially occlude (as if they were strangled by one hand) and this considerably slows the return of venous blood to the heart. As a consequence, the arterial pressure rises, reaching even impressive values such as 300 mmHg (usually 120 mmHg at rest). Moreover, as a consequence of the reduced blood supply to the heart, the outgoing blood also slows down and reduces, which decreases the blood and oxygen supply to the peripheral organs. Less blood and oxygen to the brain could result in dizziness, blurred vision, etc. until you eventually faint. These are side effects well-known by opera singers who practice hyperventilation exercises that, in some parts, are performed in apnoea.

Chapter 3: Machines or Free Weights?

The question is interesting, and the purpose of this chapter is to precisely evaluate the advantages and disadvantages of two possible training solutions for muscle strengthening: the use of gym machines or exercise with the aid of free weights.

From a health point of view, it is clear that the question of the title seems reasonable because, unlike in a bodybuilder, muscle strengthening is seen only as a preparatory to a sport or as a general improvement of the body, and therefore it is not said that the use of gym machines is actually the only possible solution for those who want to make a good upgrade without wanting to reach professional levels of a bodybuilding lover. Before analyzing the two solutions in detail, briefly remember that a muscle can perform an effort in two ways of contraction: eccentric or concentric.

In the first case, the muscle develops the force necessary for the exercise when it is stretching, in the second case when it is being shortened.

Weights and machines are not always equivalent in stimulating a muscle in an eccentric and concentric way. For the purpose of training, eccentric work is the most difficult—to the point that it can also induce pain and muscle damage. It is therefore important that, by deciding which exercises to perform (with the machines or with the weights), it is clear (otherwise you can ask the instructor like I did at the beginning of my journey in the gym) which exercises stimulate the muscles more eccentrically, to introduce them gradually into the plan of training avoiding injuries.

Weight Machines

In the gym, there are usually many weight machines. Generally, except for the multi-function stations, each of them trains a specific muscular district or even a single type of muscle. The effort put in place by the muscles during the execution of the exercise must counteract two physical forces: the weight force and the force due to the friction of the weight that it moves (often along ropes or pulleys).

As a general rule of the mechanics involved in the use of weights, during the eccentric contraction, the friction force is subtracted from that of the weight, while during the concentric contraction this force is added.

Free Weights

They are called free-weight exercises because usually the weights are not tied to ropes or pulleys of the machines, but simply gripped or tied to the body (for example with anklets) and carried out only with the aid of weights such as dumbbells and barbells, which are often seen on sale in supermarkets. Surely, compared to a workout with machines, the one with free weights is easier to put in place. Often, it is not even necessary to attend a gym; a small home space equipped with a mat, a bench (if required by the exercises), a mirror (optional, to control the movements) and, of course, the weights is sufficient enough.

Now let's analyze the advantages and disadvantages of the two solutions, taking into consideration some objective parameters that can assume different importance depending on the individual's objectives, the physical state of departure (sedentary, beginner or advanced athlete), and the expectations placed in a training of this type.

Economic aspect: free weight training is certainly cheaper, because, as mentioned, in most cases it is not necessary to get a gym subscription. It can be a good compromise solution to go to the gym for the time necessary to practice the exercises under the guidance of an experienced instructor, and then, once you are sure to perform the correct movements, buy weights and equip yourself with a training-space inside your home. This is what I did, and I would never go back.

Versatility: free weights are suitable for multiple exercises and different muscle groups. Think about how many exercises you can do with simple weights to train biceps, triceps, pectorals, etc. In the case of training with weight machines, each machine usually allows a few exercises (if not only one) and this is the practical limit of such a training: you need to choose a gym where there is a sufficient number of machines for the exercises you want to do and where waiting times are not too long. Otherwise, the queues to the machines make the overall workout boring and ineffective.

Eccentric and concentric training: weight machines usually lesser stress the eccentric work of the muscle (because of the opposing frictional force) unlike the movement of the body which, in returning to the starting position of the exercise, often performs eccentric work of considerable intensity. Moreover, in the exercises with weights, many antagonistic muscles are trained many times, and in general, they also train the balance and proprioceptive, improving body coordination.

Safety and complexity: from the previous point, we can see that weight machines train specific muscle areas, and it is easier to isolate the muscle or muscle district involved. It is also easier to perform the exercise correctly because the movements are constrained by the machines and are easier to learn. With free weights, it is easier to make mistakes, and generally more antagonistic muscles and the spine are stimulated. In addition, with the weights, it is easier to maintain a constant execution speed. For all these reasons, it is generally said that the exercises with the machines are at a lower risk of injury than those with free weights.

Chapter 4: Putting it all together. How to program a training cycle

Now we come to the crucial point: how do I craft a strength training program? The question is very complex. Each strategy will be based on the condition of the subject, so, logically, when we see a disproportionate lack of strength for a muscle group, it will be logical to intervene in this sense. Let's go step by step. The literature on the subject highlights how, for the purposes of muscular hypertrophy and gains in strength, setting a periodized program is the best solution. Before diving deeper into the topic, it is important to note something. You cannot generalize, there is no way to use a unique approach or way of training a particular component. There are countless cases, solutions. So what can be done is to report different models based on different contexts to give not a guide but a concept—something infinitely more precious (and expendable).

Strategy 1. "Basic" Approach. A first approach that we can use is to set up a multifrequency workout by adopting a daily wavy periodization. So we will have two weekly sessions for each muscle district. In the first session we can train the muscle according to a traditional bodybuilding scheme, then longer TUT, intensity techniques, a range of 8-12 repetitions, eccentric, forced, etc. In the second session, we can train ourselves by adopting a progression of strength. So for example, we will train the chest on a flat bench using possibly another complementary exercise (like crosses, chest fly, etc.). A similar approach is at the base of the PHAT (Power Hypertrophy Adaptive Training) method proposed by Norton. Unlike this, however, I find it more sensible to use—in training dedicated to strength—real progressions on exercises without being limited to a 5 × 5 standard type of training.

Strategy 2. Deficient Muscles Approach. Similar to the previous one, the only difference is that a workout in this sense will be done on the deficient muscles while the more developed muscles will be trained in mono-frequency. The increase in weekly volume and stimulus variation will bring an advantage in terms of growth (strength and hypertrophy) that will allow you to "catch up" with respect to the rest of the muscles. This approach can be used on deficient muscles both from a hypertrophy point of view and from a force point of view (i.e., the weakest muscles). This last aspect is particularly important as it can be a valid strategy to intervene where a muscle is placed limiting within the synergy of a gesture. The discourse can also be done from the opposite point of view—that is, to hold the strongest or most developed muscle groups to a multifrequency and to mono-frequency to recover asymmetries (aesthetic or functional).

Strategy 3. The transient phase of reduced volume. Another way to insert a strength training within a bodybuilding program is to provide a period with a high load intensity and a reduced volume. In this case, we always speak of wavy periodization. However, the variations will not be done on a daily basis, but weekly. So, for instance, we will put 2-3 up to 6 weeks of strength training with a reduced volume—less dense workouts but with the intensity of high-load and then return, progressively or not, to traditional bodybuilding sessions, or even to a wavy periodization protocol on a daily basis as described above. Basically, it is a matter of setting a transitional phase aimed at two purposes: Varying the stimulus (Ri) and finding the feeling with the motor scheme.

Strategy 4. Periodization within the session. This is also an interesting approach. It is a matter of inserting, within the session, an exercise on which to set up a forced schedule. In this sense, we could then insert the flat bench into a chest session as a first or second exercise. We will choose a program to improve on strength (since we are already able to exercise the right mastery over the exercise) and set the rest of the session as a traditional bodybuilding session. Obviously, the total volume will decrease as part of the session is occupied by dense work—not very voluminous but very intense. I find that such a setting fits well with the daily wavy periodization (strategy 1). Basically, by training a multi-frequency muscle, we will set the strength session using an exercise with its progression and the rest of the session in the traditional bodybuilding style. The diversification of work with respect to the second weekly session will be in the TUT (for example) which, in the latter, will be exasperated (e.g., +50'), while in the session of "strength" it will not be too high (e.g., 30').

Split and choice of exercises

A further aspect on which we must dwell is that relative to the decision, within the session, the target muscle groups and the exercises to be used. One of the characteristics of strength programs is that, in most cases, the various muscle groups are subdivided to work only a few each session. This is logical because the work that is required is always of the same type (anaerobic). Okay, as we have seen, it can work on different adaptive components, but in any case, it is always part of the big family of "boosting" work, the same that, in other sports, is alternated with "technical" work. The question that arises is the following: Should we first set the split and then, based on this, choose the type of exercises in which to work the strength or vice versa? Being a powerlifter myself, I would answer "the second," but from a Bodybuilder perspective I would answer "the first." Since this chapter is about strength training, I would say start from this context and, in particular, from the cases mentioned above. Where we want to set a wavy periodization, for all groups or only for some (strategies 1-2-4), then yes, we will have to start from the split. Based on this we will choose the best exercise on which to progress for the strength. So for example, in a push-day, we will choose the Bench Press for the chest, for a pull-day a Bent Over Row, and for a leg-day a Squat.

Let's do an example: Subject 1, Powerlifter, good management of high loads on the various motor schemes. Deficient groups: Arms, Back. Strong groups: Chest, Quadriceps

Split

Day 1 Push Day

Day 2 Pull Day

Day 3 Leg Day

Day 4 Rest

Day 5 Arms

Day 6 Back

Day 7 Glutes

Logically, we will then insert a progression on the Bent-Over Row on day 2 and work the Back with a traditional strength session on day 6. To evaluate a progression on the ground clearance that would be close to a leg workout (even putting it on day 6), we will have the hamstrings on day 7. But training strength, as we have seen, is not just a matter of periodizing and varying the stimulus, but also a question of functionality to the motor schemes to be performed during the sessions.

So let's take another example. Subject 2: Powerlifter, poor activation of the chest on the bench press, poor feeling on the deadlift. Excellent management of the

Squat. Deficient groups: Chest-Back-Arms. The goal, in this case, will be to improve the feeling with easier exercises so we will set the split based on the same.

Split

Day 1 Chest and Shoulders

Day 2 Deadlift day

Day 3 Rest

Day 4 Quadriceps and Arms

Day 5 Rest

Day 6 Chest and Back

Day 7 Arms

Finally, in case we go set up a Strength program as a transitory phase (strategy 3), it will be logical to start from the exercises and, based on these, reason on the split.

PART 4

Chapter 1: What Is the Ketogenic Diet

In this first chapter, we are going to discuss what the ketogenic diet is and why it is becoming more and more popular these days. In fact, you can browse the web for a few minutes, and you will easily find articles and blogs dedicated to this topic. Most people, however, decide to follow the diet without actually knowing what they are getting themselves into and are not able to distinguish good information from harmful ones. This is why we decided to start off the book by laying out the foundation of this diet, so everybody will understand its principles. Let us get started!

If there is a diet that is often misunderstood it is the ketogenic diet. Publicized by some as a very effective means of weight loss, criticized by others for the supposed — and often exaggerated — risks associated with it. It is actually an important tool, especially when it comes to improving one's health. Any particular diet that must be used with due precautions, but the keto diet can guarantee effective results where other methods often fail.

The idea on which the ketogenic diet is based is the ability of our body to use lipid reserves with great effectiveness when the availability of carbohydrates is greatly reduced. The physiological mechanisms activated in this situation reduce the possible use of proteins for energy, protecting the lean mass and significantly reducing the sensation of hunger.

In the clinical field, the first documented use of a ketogenic diet to treat specific diseases dates back to the 1920s when Russell Wilder used it to control attacks in pediatric patients with epilepsy that could not be treated with drugs. The keto diet became the center of attention again in the 1990s, and since then, the usage of the diet increased. In the 60s and 70s, with the constant increase of obesity among the populace, numerous studies were carried out on the use of a low-calorie diet that could lead to rapid and significant weight reduction without affecting the lean mass.

The various protocols of PSMF (Protein Sparing Modified Fast) were born, these are diets characterized by a reduced protein intake with a near-total absence of carbohydrates and a measured protein intake aimed at minimizing the loss of precious muscle mass. The implementation of the ketogenic diet saw a surge with the appearance of low-carb diets and do-it-yourself diets on the market, such as the Atkins diet. Although, that is a shameful model that drastically reduces the consumption of carbohydrates instead so one can freely eat fat and proteins. The Atkins diet is a grotesque caricature of the ketogenic diet based on improbable and fanciful interpretations of human physiology, which is why it was rightly criticized by the entire scientific community.

Recently, the emergence of the Paleo diet has brought attention back to food regimens that emphasize reduced carbohydrate content to generate ketosis. Here, solid scientific basis intertwines with perturbed, poorly-engineered biological concepts that have often generated ineffective solutions where every carbohydrate is disregarded and considered a poison, while the consumption of bacon is recommended, as it was the staple diet during the Paleolithic era. Now, there has been a renewed interest within the scientific community towards this diet, starting with the investigation on the use of the ketogenic diet for the treatment of obesity and other medical conditions or issues such as the formation of tumors, neurological diseases like Alzheimer's and Parkinson's disease, diabetes, and metabolic syndrome as well.

The human body has several ways to accumulate energy reserves, the most consistent of which is through the use of adipose tissue (fat). An average individual weighing 70 kg, can have as much as 15 kg of adipose tissue, while the carbohydrate portion amounts to little less than half a kilogram. It is evident that sugar reserves can guarantee energy for very limited periods of time, while fats represent a huge reserve of energy. Tissues receive energy in proportion to the actual availability of substrates in the blood. When glucose is present in sufficient quantities, it appears to be the most preferred energy source used by all of the body's tissues. When glucose is in short supply, most organs and tissues can use fatty acids as an energy source, or they convert other substances into sugars, especially some amino acids like alanine and glutamine, through a process called gluconeogenesis.

Some organs and tissues like the brain, central nervous system, red blood cells, and type II muscle fibers cannot use free fatty acids. But, when the body experiences glucose deficiency, they can use ketone bodies. These are substances derived from lipidic parts, the concentration of which is usually very small under normal conditions but increase considerably in particular situations, such as a prolonged fasting or a long period without carbohydrate consumption.

The increase in the concentration of ketone bodies in the blood, resulting from fasting or severe reduction of their food intake with the diet, is a completely natural condition called ketosis. This is a mechanism that was developed to help us cope with the stringent metabolic needs and limited availability of food back when our ancestors lived in a hunter-gatherer society. This process also naturally occurs in the morning after fasting overnight or after an intense and vigorous physical activity.

The severe restriction of carbohydrate intake through the action of hormones such as insulin and glucagon promotes the mobilization of lipids from the reserve tissues and their use as fuel. Given the scarcity of glucose, the present Acetyl-CoA is used for the production of ketone bodies while substances such as acetone, acetoacetate, and β-hydroxybutyric acid, become the preferred fuel for the cells of the

central nervous system. During ketosis, blood sugar is maintained at normal levels thanks to the presence of glucogenic amino acids and, above all, glycerol, which is derived from the demolition of triglycerides for the formation of glucose.

In physiological ketosis, the presence of ketone bodies in the blood passes from 0.1 mmol/dl to about 7 mmol/dl. The significant alteration of the body's pH levels, which normally stays around 7.4 but could decrease slightly in the first few days given the acidity of ketone bodies, may return quickly to normal levels as long as the concentration of ketone bodies remains below 10 mmol/dl.

The effect of saving protein reserves could occur through different mechanisms which is why the use of proteins is important during the first few days of the diet. But, as the body begins to predominantly use free fatty acids and ketones for their energy needs, the demand for glucose drops drastically, accompanied by the reduction of the use of amino acids for energy purposes. A direct effect of the ketone bodies on protein metabolism and on the functions of the thyroid is not excluded, a noticeable effect is the reduction of T3.

The excess ketones are eliminated through breathing in the form of acetone, which induces what we refer to as 'acetone breath,' and through the urine, where excess acidity is buffered by simultaneous elimination of sodium, potassium, and magnesium.

Ketosis introduces changes in the concentration of different hormones and nutrients, including ghrelin, amylin, leptin and, of course, ketone bodies themselves. It is probably through these variations that one of the most relevant effects of the ketogenic diet is initiated: the reduction or total disappearance of the sensation of hunger. This is undoubtedly a situation that better helps one to endure the typical rigor of this diet.

Chapter 2: The Three Principles of the Ketogenic Diet

The ketogenic diet is based on 3 essential concepts:

Reduction of simple and complex carbohydrates

Foods containing carbohydrates must be totally eliminated, even if this is practically impossible. The portions of the vegetables which contain fructose are maintained, resulting in the collapse of complex carbohydrates in favor of the simple ones which are very low in quantity. These nutrients are used as a primary energy source by most organisms. When they're reduced to a minimum, the body is then forced to dispose of excess fat reserves. Moreover, carbohydrates are nutrients that significantly stimulate insulin (anabolic and fattening hormones), so their moderation should also have metabolic significance.

Partial increase of fats and a percentage of proteins to keep the increase of calories constant

After eliminating the carbohydrates, consumption of protein-rich foods should be kept constant, as well as foods with a high content of fats (oils, oil seeds, oily fleshy fruits, etc.). In theory, this compensates for the caloric reduction of glucose thanks to the greater quantity of lipids. In practice, for obvious reasons like appetite (or hunger), it is necessary to increase the portions and frequency of the consumption of protein sources.

Some justify this 'correction' by stating that more proteins are useful for conserving lean mass. It should be specified, however, that many amino acids are glucogenic (they are converted into glucose by neoglucogenesis) and have a metabolic action similar to carbohydrates, partially negating the effect on lipolytic enzymes and lessening the production of ketone bodies (see below). Moreover, in clinical practice, the menu of the ketogenic diet is never normocaloric and provides less energy than necessary. Which is why, before you venture into such a strict regimen, you should try a well-balanced calorie

diet first.

Production of ketone bodies

The hepatic neoglucogenesis necessary to synthesize glucose (starting from certain amino acids and glycerol) is not fast enough to cover the daily glucose needs of the body. At the same time, fat oxidation (closely related to and dependent on glycolysis) 'jams' and causes the accumulation of intermediate molecules called ketone bodies. These ketones, which at physiological concentrations are easily disposable, in the ketogenic diet reach levels that are toxic for the tissues.

Toxic does not necessarily mean poisonous, but rather, it is something which causes intoxication. This effect is clearly distinguishable by the reduction of appetite, that is, the anorectic effect on the brain. Although, like the heart, the nervous tissue can partially use the ketone bodies to generate energy.

A healthy organism can function with high quantities of ketone bodies in the blood since the excess is eliminated (we do not know how much effort is required by the body to accomplish this) through renal filtration. Obviously, people suffering from certain pathologies (defects in insulin secretion that's typical of type 1 diabetes, renal failure which is also triggered by advanced type 2 diabetes, liver failure, etc.) have a very high risk of developing metabolic acidosis or diabetic ketoacidosis, risking coma or even death.

Chapter 3: An Example of the Ketogenic Diet Meal Plan

Now it is time to dive right into the core of the ketogenic diet. Here are some of the meals that you can try to start off with:

Breakfast

A protein source:

- o Eggs
- o 50 g of meat preserved as bacon, raw ham, or bresaola

25 - 50 g of carbohydrates

- o Rye bread
- o Dried fruit
- o Pistachios
- o Peanuts
- o Peanut butter

30g of fat

- o Low-carbohydrate and high-fat cheese
- o Flakes
- o Milk

     o   Butter

Mid-morning snack

A mid-morning snack can provide a modest intake of carbohydrates that can be taken from these choices

     Two teaspoons of peanut butter and celery

     50g of dried fruit

     Toasted pistachios

     Almonds

   Toasted peanuts

Lunch

During the week, lunch can take the form of the any of the following:

     A protein source of about 200 - 250 g: o

       Fish like salmon or trout or tuna o

       Meat like chicken or turkey

          A portion of 100 - 200 g of vegetables:

     o   Salad

     o   Green beans

     o   Salad rocket

- o   Lettuce

- o   Asparagus

- o   Mushrooms

- o   Broccoli

- o   Peas

A source of fat of about 25g:

- o   Olive oil

- o   Butter

- o   Mayonnaise

- o   Cream

Mid-afternoon snack

Alternate the following foods during the week:

A source of fat, around 50 - 100

g: o   Cheese

- o   Flakes

- o   Milk

A protein source or a modest source of

carbohydrates: o   Vegetable soup

- o   Carrots

- o   Peas

Dinner

During the week, dinner can be eaten through any of the following:

A protein source of about 150 - 200 g:

- o   Meat such as hamburger, veal, or goat
- o   Fish such as trout, salmon, tuna, or swordfish
- o   Eggs

A source of fat of around 20 - 30 g:

- o   Cheese
- o   Oil
- o   Butter
- o   Bacon

A portion of vegetables of about 200 g:

- o   Salad
- o   String beans
- o   Rocket salad
- o   Lettuce
- o   Asparagus
- o   Mushrooms
- o   Broccoli
- o   Tomatoes

o   Peppers

o   Peas

Chapter 4: Two Types of Ketogenic Diet

There are two main types of ketogenic diet: the intermittent ketogenic diet and the cyclic ketogenic diet. There is also a whole series of diets that follow the same basic principle of the ketogenic diet, which is weight loss obtained through the action of the ketogenic bodies. In this final chapter, we will take a look at the

two main types of ketogenic diet.

Cyclic ketogenic diet

It is the most widely used type of ketogenic diet, and it is divided into two different phases. The first phase lasts about 5 - 6 days and includes a low-carbohydrate intake in the diet, as well as a recharging phase that has a duration of 1 - 2 days, which requires carbohydrate consumption to be very high. In this way, the muscle glycogen reserves are replenished for a whole week during the refill phase. In the second phase, 10 - 12 grams of carbohydrates per kg of body weight must be consumed each and every day.

Intermittent ketogenic diet

This ketogenic diet is a type of diet followed a lot by athletes in general, but not by those who practice sports like bodybuilding, in which the activity is aimed at increasing muscle mass. In this diet, the body supplies muscle glycogen stores, which makes it suitable for those who practice aerobic exercises. The carbohydrate refilling phase takes place during the entire week, and each meal is recommended to provide at least 0.7 g of carbohydrates for every kilogram of body weight.

PART 5

CHAPTER 1: KETO BASICS

BENEFITS OF INCREASED METABOLISM

One of the best ways to learn the meaning of a scientific term is to break it down to its roots. When we break down ketogenic, we see it is comprised of two words: keto and genic. Ketones are fat-based molecules that the body breaks down when it is using fat as its energy source. When used as a suffix, "genic" means "causing, forming, or producing." So, we put these terms together, and we have "ketogenic," or simply put, "causing fat burn." Ergo, the theory behind ketogenic dieting is: when a person reduces the amount of sugar and carbohydrates they consume, the body will begin to breakdown fat it already has in stores all over the body. When your body is cashing in on these stores, it is in a ketogenic state, or "ketosis." When your body consumes food, it naturally seeks carbohydrates for the purpose of breaking them down and using them as fuel. Adversely, a ketogenic cleanse trains your body to use fats for energy instead. This is achieved by lowering the amount of ingested carbohydrates and increasing the amount of ingested fats, which in turn boosts your metabolism.

Only recently has a low carb- high-fat diet plan emerged into the public eye. It is a sharp contrast to the traditional dieting style that emphasizes calorie counting. For many years it was overlooked that crash diets neglect the most important aspect of dieting: food is fuel. A diet is not meant to be treated as a once a year go to method in order to shed holiday weight in January. Rather, a diet is a lifestyle; it is a consistent pattern of how individual fuels their body. A ten day ketogenic cleanse is the perfect way to begin forming healthy eating habits that over time become second nature. If you are tired of losing weight just to gain it all back, never fear. We firmly believe that you can accomplish anything you put your mind to, including living a healthy life! You, like hundreds of others, can successfully accomplish a ketogenic cleanse and change the way you see health, fitness, and life along the way. So let's hit the books and get that metabolism working!

BENEFITS OF CLEANSING

In addition to increased metabolism and fat loss, ketogenic cleansing allows your body naturally rid itself of harmful toxins and wasteful substances. In today's modern world, food is overrun and polluted by genetically modified hormones, artificial flavors and coloring, and copious amounts of unnecessary sugars. Ketogenic cleansing eliminates bread, grains, and many other foods that are most affected by today's modern industrialization. Due to the high amount of naturally occurring foods used in a ketogenic cleanse, the body is able to obtain many vitamins and minerals that are not prevalent in a high carb diet. When the body is consuming sufficient amounts of necessary vitamins and minerals, it is able to heal itself and maintain a healthy immune system. Cleansing your body is one of the best ways to achieve, and maintain pristine health.

CHAPTER 2: MEAL PLAN MADNESS

One of the best ways to stay motivated, when dieting, is to find a meal plan that is easy to follow and easy on the budget. Ketogenic meals are designed to be filling while keeping within the perimeters of low-carb, high-fat guidelines. Ideally, you want to aim for 70% fats, 25% protein, and 5% carbohydrates in your diet. As long as the materials you use to build your meals are low in carbs and high in fats, feel free to experiment and find what is right for you. Each and every one of us is different, and that's okay. After all, this meal plan is for YOU!

Below is a ten-day meal plan, designed with a busy schedule in mind, which will not break the bank! All of these meals can be prepared in 30 minutes or less, and many of them are much quicker than that! There is also a list of ingredients for each meal located in the recipe chapter so you can go to the grocery store knowing exactly what you need!

	Breakfast	Lunch	Dinner
Day 1	California Chicken Omelet Fat: 32 grams 10 minutes to prepare Protein: 25 grams 10	Cobb Salad Fat: 48 grams 10 minutes to prepare Protein: 43 grams 0 minutes of cooking Net carbs: 3 grams	Chicken Peanut Pad Thai Fat: 12 grams 15 minutes to prepare Protein: 30 grams 15 minutes of cooking Net carbs: 2 grams

	minutes of cooking Net carbs: 4 grams		
Day 2	**Easy Blender Pancakes** Fat: 29 grams 5 minutes to prepare Protein: 41 grams 10 minutes of cooking Net carbs: 4 grams	**Sardine Stuffed Avocados** Fat: 29 grams 10 minutes to prepare Protein: 27 grams 0 minutes of cooking Net Carbs: 5 grams	**Chipotle Fish Tacos** Fat: 20 grams 5 minutes to prepare Protein: 24 grams 15 minutes of cooking Net carbs: 5 grams
Day 3	**Steak and Eggs** Fat: 36 grams 10 minutes to prepare Protein: 47 grams 5 minutes of cooking Net carbs: 3 grams	**Low-Carb Smoothie Bowl** Fat 35 grams 5 minutes to prepare Protein: 20 grams 0 minutes of cooking Net carbs: 5 grams	**Avocado Lime Salmon** Fat: 27 grams 20 minutes to prepare Protein: 37 grams 10 minutes of cooking Net carbs: 5 grams
KEEP IT UP!!!	During the course of your plan, especially around days 3 and 4, you may begin to feel like you don't have it in you. You may have thoughts telling you that you cannot last for ten days on this type pf cleanse. Do not allow feelings of discouragement bother you because guess what?		

	We all feel that way sometimes! A ketogenic diet causes your body to process energy like it never has before. Keep pressing on! Your body will thank you and so will you!		
Day 4	**Low-Carb Smoothie Bowl** Fat: 35 grams 5 minutes to prepare Protein: 35 grams 0 minutes of cooking Net carbs: 4 grams	**Pesto Chicken Salad** Fat: 27 grams 5 minutes to prepare Protein: 27 grams 10 minutes of cooking Net carbs: 3 grams	**Sriracha Lime Flank Steak** Fat: 32 grams 5 minutes to prepare Protein: 48 grams 10 minutes of cooking Net Carbs: 5 grams
Day 5	**Feta and Pesto Omelet** Fat: 46 grams 5 minutes of preparation Protein: 30 grams 5 minutes of cooking Net carbs: 2.5 grams	**Roasted Brussel Sprouts** Fat: 21 grams 5 minutes to prepare Protein: 21 grams 30 minutes of cooking Net carbs: 4 grams	**Low carb Sesame Chicken** Fat: 36 grams 15 minutes to prepare Protein: 41 grams 15 minutes of cooking Net carbs: 4 grams
Day 6	**Raspberry Cream Crepes** Fat: 40 grams 5 minutes of preparation Net carbs: 8 grams 15 minutes of cooking	**Shakshuka** Fat: 34 grams Protein 35 grams Net carbs: 4	**Sausage in a Pan** Fat: 38 grams 10 minutes of preparation

	Protein 15 grams	grams 10 minutes of preparation 10 minutes of cooking	Protein: 30 grams 25 minutes of cooking Net Carbs: 4 grams
Day 7	**Green Monster Smoothie** Fat: 25 grams 5 minutes of preparation Protein: 30 grams 0 minutes of cooking Net Carbs: 3 grams	**Tuna Tartare** Fat: 24 grams 15 minutes of preparation Protein: 56 grams 0 minutes of cooking Net Carbs: 4 grams	**Pesto Chicken Salad** Fat: 27 grams 5 minutes of preparation Protein: 27 grams 10 minutes of cooking Net carbs: 3 grams
ALMO ST THER E!!	By now, you can be certain you are seeing physical results such as reduced body fat and more energy! You are doing a fantastic job, and you only have three days left! Keep up the good work; you owe it to yourself.		
Day 8	**Shakshuka** Fat: 34 grams 10 minutes of preparation Protein 35 grams 10 minutes	**Grilled Halloumi Salad** Fat: 47 grams 15 minutes of preparation Protein: 21 grams 0 minutes of cooking Net carbs: 2 grams	**Keto Quarter Pounder** Fat: 34 grams 10 minutes of preparation Protein: 25 grams 8

	of cooking Net carbs: 4 grams		minutes of cooking Net carbs: 4
Day 9	**Easy Blender Pancakes** Fat: 29 grams 5 minutes of preparation Protein: 41 grams 10 minutes of cooking Net carbs: 4 grams	**Broccoli Bacon Salad** Fat: 31 grams 15 minutes of preparation Protein: 10 grams 6 minutes of cooking Net carbs: 5 grams	**Sardine Stuffed Avocados** Fat: 29 grams 10 minutes to prepare Protein: 27 grams 0 minutes to cook Net Carbs: 5 grams
Day 10	**California Chicken Omelet** Fat 32 grams 10 minutes to prepare Protein 25 grams 10 minutes of cooking Net Carb: 3 grams	**Shrimp Scampi** Fat: 21 grams 5 minutes to prepare Protein: 21 grams 30 minutes of cooking Net carbs: 4 grams	**Tuna Tartare** Fat: 36 grams 15 minutes to prepare Protein: 41 grams 15 minutes of cooking Net carbs: 4 grams
YOU DID	Congratulations! You have successfully completed a 10 day ketogenic cleanse. By now your body has adjusted to its new source of energy,		

IT!!	expelled dozens of harmful toxins, and replenished itself with many vitamins and minerals it may have been lacking. Way to go on a job well done!

CHAPTER 3: BREAKFAST IS FOR CHAMPIONS

Breakfast is by far the most important meal of the day for one reason: it set the tone for the rest of your day. In order to hit the ground running, it is vital that one starts each day with foods that fuel an energetic and productive day. This chapter contains ten ketogenic breakfast ideas that will have you burning fat and conquering your day like you never imagined.

1. CALIFORNIA CHICKEN OMELET

This recipe requires 10 minutes of preparation, 10 minutes of cooking time and serves 1

Net carbs: 4 grams

Protein: 25 grams

Fat : 32 grams

What you will need:

- Mayo (1 tablespoon)

- Mustard (1 teaspoon)

- Campari tomato

- Eggs (2 large beaten)

- Avocado (one-fourth, sliced)

- Bacon (2 slices cooked and chopped)

- Deli chicken (1 ounce)

What to do:

1. Place a skillet on the stove over a burner set to a medium heat and let it warm before adding the eggs and seasoning as needed.

2. Once eggs are cooked about halfway through, add bacon, chicken, avocado, tomato, mayo, and mustard on one side of the eggs.

3. Fold the omelet onto its self, cover and cook for 5 additional minutes.

4. Once eggs are fully cooked, and all ingredients are warm, through the center, your omelet is ready.

5. Bon apatite!

2. STEAK AND EGGS WITH AVOCADO

This recipe requires 10 minutes of preparation, 5 minutes of cooking time and serves 1

Net Carbs: 3 grams

Protein: 44 grams

Fat: 36 grams

What you will need:

- Salt and pepper

- Avocado (one-fourth, sliced)

- Sirloin steak (4 ounces)

- Eggs (3 large)

- Butter (1 tablespoon)

What to do:

1. Melt the tablespoon of butter in a pan and fry all 3 eggs to the desired doneness. Season the eggs with salt and pepper.

2. In a different pan, cook the sirloin steak to your preferred taste and slice it into thin strips. Season the steak with salt and pepper.

3. Sever your prepared steak and eggs with slices of avocado.

4. Enjoy!

3. PANCAKES IN A BLENDER

This recipe requires 5 minutes of preparation, 10 minutes of cooking time and serves 1

Net Carbs: 4 grams

Protein: 41 grams

Fat: 29 grams

What you will need:

- Whey protein powder (1 scoop) -

Eggs (2 large)

- Cream cheese (2 ounces)

- Just a pinch of cinnamon and a pinch of salt

What to do:

1. Combine cream cheese, eggs, protein powder, cinnamon, and salt in a blender. Blend for 10 seconds and let stand.

2. While letting batter stand, warm a skillet over medium heat.

3. Pour about ¼ of the batter into warmed skillet and let cook. When bubbles begin to emerge on the surface, flip the pancake.

4. Once flipped, cook for 15 seconds. Repeat until the remainder of the batter is used up.

5. Top with butter and/ or sugar- free maple syrup and you are all set!

6. Chow time!

4. LOW CARB SMOOTHE BOWL

Net Carbs: 4 grams

Protein: 35 grams

Fat: 35 grams

It takes 5 minutes to prepare and serves 1.

What you will need:

- Spinach (1 cup)

- Almond milk (half a cup) -

Coconut oil (1 tablespoon)

- Low carb protein powder (1 scoop) -

Ice cubes (2 cubes)

- Whipping cream (2 T)

- Optional toppings can include: raspberries, walnuts, shredded coconut, or chia seeds

What to do:

1. Place spinach in the blender. Add almond milk, cream, coconut oil, and ice. Blend until thoroughly and evenly combined.

2. Pour into bowl.

3. Top with toppings or stir lightly into a smoothie.

4. Treat yourself!

5. FETA AND PESTO OMELET

This recipe requires 5 minutes of preparation, 5 minutes of cooking time and serves 1

Net Carbs: 2.5 grams

Protein: 30 grams

Fat: 46 grams

What you will need:

- Butter (1 tablespoon)

- Eggs (3 large)

- Heavy cream (1 tablespoon)

- Feta cheese (1 ounce)

- Basil pesto (1 teaspoon)

- Tomatoes (optional)

What to do:

1. Heat pan and melt butter.

2. Beat eggs together with heavy whipping cream (will give eggs a fluffy consistency once cooked).

3. Pour eggs into pan and cook until almost done, add feta and pesto to on half of the eggs.

4. Fold omelet and cook for an additional 4-5 minutes.

5. Top with feta and tomatoes, and eat up!

6. CREPES WITH CREAM AND RASPBERRIES

This recipe requires 5 minutes of preparation, 15 minutes of cooking time and serves 2

Net Carbs: 8 grams

Protein: 15 grams

Fat: 40 grams

What you will need:

- Raspberries (3 ounces, fresh or frozen)

- Whole Milk Ricotta (half a cup and 2 tablespoons)

- Erythritol (2 tablespoons)

- Eggs (2 large)

- Cream Cheese (2 ounces)

- Pinch of salt

- Dash of Cinnamon

- Whipped cream and sugar- free maple syrup to go on

top What to do:

1. In a blender, blend cream cheese, eggs, erythritol, salt, and cinnamon for about 20 seconds, or until there are no lumps of cream cheese.

2. Place a pan on a burner turned to a medium heat before coating in cooking spray. Add 20 percent of your batter to the pan in a thin layer. Cook crepe until the underside becomes slightly darkened. Carefully flip the crepe and let the reverse side cook for about 15 seconds.

3. Repeat step 3 until all batter is used.

4. Without stacking the crepes, allow them to cool for a few minutes.

5. After the crepes have cool, place about 2 tablespoons of ricotta cheese in the center of each crepe.

6. Throw in a couple of raspberries and fold the side to the middle.

7. Top those off with some whipped cream and sugar- free maple syrup and…

8. Viola! You're a true chef! Indulge in your creation!

7. GREEN MONSTER SMOOTHIE

This recipe requires 10 minutes of preparation, 0 minutes of cooking time and serves 1

Net Carbs: 4 grams

Protein: 30 grams

Fat: 25 grams

What you will need:

- Almond milk (one and a half cups)

- Spinach (one-eighth of a cup)

- Cucumber (a fourth of a cup)

- Celery (a fourth of a cup)

- Avocado (a fourth of a cup)

- Coconut oil (1 tablespoon)

- Stevia (liquid, 10 drops)

- Whey Protein Powder (1

scoop) What to do:

1. In a blender, blend almond milk and spinach for a few pulses.

2. Add remaining ingredients and blend until thoroughly combined.

3. Add optional matcha powder, if desired, and enjoy!

CHAPTER 4: LUNCH CRUNCH

Eating a healthy lunch when you are limited on time due to, work, school, or taking care of your kids can be a tumultuous task. Thankfully, we have compiled a list of eight quick and easy recipes to accompany the ten-day meal plan laid out in chapter 2! Many find it advantageous, especially if you work throughout the week, to prepare your meals ahead of time. Thankfully, these lunch recipes are also easy to pack and take on the go!

1. OFF THE COBB SALAD

Net carbs: 3 grams

Protein: 43 grams

Fat: 48 grams

It takes 10 minutes to prepare and serves

1. What you will need:

- Spinach (1 cup)

- Egg (1, hard-boiled) -

Bacon (2 strips)

- Chicken breast (2 ounces)

- Campari tomato (one-half of tomato) -

Avocado (one-fourth, sliced)

- White vinegar (half of a teaspoon) -

Olive oil (1 tablespoon)

What to do:

1. Cook chicken and bacon completely and cut or slice into small pieces.

2. Chop remaining ingredients into bite size pieces.

3. Place all ingredients, including chicken and bacon, in a bowl, toss ingredients in oil and vinegar.

4. Enjoy!

2. AVOCADO AND SARDINES

Net Carbs: 5 grams

Protein: 27 grams

Fat: 52 grams

It takes 10 minutes to prepare and serves

1. What you will need:

- Fresh lemon juice (1 tablespoon)

- Spring onion or chives (1 or small bunch) -

Mayonnaise (1 tablespoon)

- Sardines (1 tin, drained)

- Avocado (1 whole, seed removed)

- Turmeric powder (a fourth of a teaspoon) or freshly ground turmeric

  root (1 teaspoon)

- Salt (a fourth of a teaspoon)

What to do:

1. Begin by cutting the avocado in half and removing its seed.

2. Scoop out about half the avocado and set aside (shown below).

3. In a small bowl, mash drained sardines with a fork.

4. Add onion (or chives), turmeric powder, and mayonnaise. Mix well.

5. Add removed avocado to sardine mixture.

6. Add lemon juice and salt.

7. Scoop the mixture into avocado halves.

8. Dig in!

3. CHICKEN SALAD A LA PESTO

This recipe requires 5minutes of preparation, 10 minutes of cooking time and serves 4

Net Carbs: 3 grams

Protein: 27 grams

Fat: 27 grams

What you will need:

- Garlic pesto (2 tablespoons)

- Mayonnaise (a fourth of a cup)

- Grape tomatoes (10, halved)

- Avocado (1, cubed)

- Bacon (6 slices, cooked crisp and crumbled)

- Chicken (1 pound, cooked and cubed)

- Romaine lettuce (optional)

What to do:

1. Combine all ingredients in a large mixing bowl.

2. Toss gently to spread mayonnaise and pesto evenly throughout.

3. If desired, wrap in romaine lettuce for a low-carb BLT chicken wrap.

4. Bon apatite!

4. BACON AND ROASTED BRUSSEL SPROUTS

This recipe requires 5 minutes of preparation, 30 minutes of cooking time and serves 4

Net Carbs: 4 grams

Protein: 15 grams

Fat: 21 grams

What you will need:

- Bacon (8 strips)
- Olive oil (2 tablespoons)
- Brussel sprouts (1 pound, halved)
- Salt and pepper

What to do:

1. Preheat oven to 375 degrees Fahrenheit.
2. Gently mix Brussel sprouts with olive oil, salt, and pepper.
3. Spread Brussel sprouts evenly onto a greased baking sheet.
4. Bake in the oven for 30 minutes. Shake the pan about halfway through to mix the Brussel sprout halves up a bit.
5. While Brussel sprouts are in the oven, fry bacon slices on the stovetop.
6. When bacon is fully cooked, let cool and chop it into bite size pieces.
7. Combine Bacon and Brussel sprouts in a bowl, and you're finished!
8. Feast!!

5. GRILLED HALLOUMI SALAD

Net Carbs: 7 grams

Protein: 21 grams

Fat: 47 grams

It takes 15 minutes to prepare and serves

1. What you will need:

- Chopped walnuts (half of an ounce) -

Baby arugula (1 handful)

- Grape tomatoes (5) -

Cucumber (1)

- Halloumi cheese (3 ounces) -

Olive oil (1 teaspoon)

- Balsamic vinegar (half of a teaspoon) -

A pinch of salt

What to do:

1. Slice halloumi cheese into slices 1/3 of an in thick.

2. Grill cheese for 3 to 5 minutes, until you see grill lines, on each side.

3. Wash and cut veggies into bite size pieces, place in salad bowl.

4. Add rinsed baby arugula and walnuts to veggies.

5. Toss in olive oil, balsamic vinegar, and salt.

6. Place grilled halloumi on top of veggies, and your lunch is ready!

7. Eat those greens and get back to work!

6. BACON BROCCOLI SALAD

This recipe requires 15 minutes of preparation, 6 minutes of cooking time and serves 5.

Net Carbs: 5 grams

Protein: 10 grams

Fat: 31 grams

What you will need:

- Sesame oil (half of a teaspoon)

- Erythritol (1 and a half tablespoons) or stevia to taste

- White vinegar (1 tablespoon)

- Mayonnaise (half of a cup)

- Green onion (three-fourths of an ounce)

- Bacon (a fourth of a pound)

- Broccoli (1 pound, heads, and stalks cut and trimmed)

What to do:

1. Cook bacon and crumble into bits.

2. Cut broccoli into bite sized pieces.

3. Slice scallions.

4. Mix mayonnaise, vinegar, erythritol (or stevia), and sesame oil, to make the dressing.

5. Place broccoli and bacon bits in a bowl and toss with dressing.

6. Viola!

7. TUNA AVOCADO TARTARE

Net Carbs: 4 grams

Protein: 56 grams

Fat: 24 grams

It takes 15 minutes to prepare and serves

2. What you will need:

- Sesame seed oil (2 tablespoons) -

Sesame seeds (1 teaspoon)

- Cucumbers (2)

- Lime (half of a whole lime) -

Mayonnaise (1 tablespoon) -

Sriracha (1 tablespoon)

- Olive oil (2 tablespoons)

- Jalapeno (one-half of the whole jalapeno) -

Scallion (3 stalks)

- Avocado (1)

- Tuna steak (1 pound)

- Soy sauce (1 tablespoon)

What to do:

1.   Dice tuna and avocado into ¼ inch cubes, place in a bowl.

2.   Finely chop scallion and jalapeno, add to bowl.

3.   Pour olive oil, sesame oil, sriracha, soy sauce, mayonnaise, and lime into a bowl.

4. Using hands, toss all ingredients to combine evenly. Using a utensil may breakdown avocado, which you want to remain chunky, so it is best to use your hands.

5. Top with sesame seeds and serve with a side of sliced cucumber.

6. There's certainly something fishy about this recipe, but it tastes great! Enjoy!

8. WARM SPINACH AND SHRIMP

This recipe requires 15 minutes of preparation, 6 minutes of cooking time and serves 5.

Fat: 24 grams

Protein: 36 grams

Net Carbs: 3 grams

Takes10 minutes to prepare, 5 minutes to cook, and serves 2.

What you will need:

- Spinach (2 handfuls)

- Parmesan (half a tablespoon)

- Heavy cream (1 tablespoon)

- Olive oil (1 tablespoon)

- Butter (2 tablespoons)

- Garlic (3 cloves)

- Onion (one fourth of whole onion)

- Large raw shrimp (about 20)

- Lemon (optional)

What to do:

1. Place peeled shrimp in cold water.

2. Chop onions and garlic into fine pieces.

3. Heat oil in a pan, over medium heat. Cook shrimp in oil until lightly pink (we do not want them fully cooked here). Remove shrimp from oil and set aside.

4. Place chopped onions and garlic into the pan, cook until onions are translucent. Add a dash of salt.

5. Add butter, cream, and parmesan cheese. Stir until you have a smooth sauce.

6. Let the sauce cook for about 2 minutes, so it will thicken slightly.

7. Place shrimp back into the pan and cook until done. This should take no longer than 2 or 3 minutes. Be careful not to overcook the shrimp; it will become dry and tough!

8. Remove shrimp and sauce from pan and replace with spinach. Cook spinach VERY briefly

9. Place warmed spinach onto a plate.

10. Pour shrimp and sauce over a bed of spinach, squeeze some lemon on top, if you like, and you're ready to chow down!

CHAPTER 5: THINNER BY DINNER

It's the end of the day and you are winding down from a hard day's work.

Your body does not require a lot of energy while you sleep; therefore, dinner

will typically consist of less fat and more protein.

1. CHICKEN PAD THAI

Net Carbs: 7 grams

Protein: 30 grams

Fat: 12 grams

It takes 15 minutes to prepare, 15 minutes to cook, and serves

4. What you will need:

- Peanuts (1 ounce) -

Lime (1 whole)

- Soy sauce (2 tablespoons) -

Egg (1 large)

- Zucchini (2 large)

- Chicken thighs (16 ounces, boneless and skinless) -

Garlic (2 cloves, minced)

- White onion (1,chopped) -

Olive oil (1 tablespoon) -

Chili flakes (optional)

What to do:

1. Over medium heat, cook olive oil and onion until translucent. Add the garlic and cook about three minutes (until fragrant).

2. Cook chicken in the pan for 5 to 7 minutes on each side (until fully cooked). Remove chicken from heat and shred it using a couple of forks.

3. Cut ends off zucchini and cut into thin noodles. Set zucchini noodles aside.

4. Next, scramble the egg in the pan.

5. Once the egg is fully cooked, and the zucchini noodles and cook for about 2 minutes.

6. Add the previously shredded chicken to the pan.

7. Give it some zing with soy sauce, lime juice, peanuts, and chili flakes.

8. Time to eat!

2. CHIPOTLE STYLE FISH TACOS

Fat: 20 grams

Protein: 24 grams

Net Carbs: 7 grams

It takes 5 minutes to prepare, 15 minutes to cook, and serves 4.

What you will need:

- Low carb tortillas (4)

- Haddock fillets (1 pound) -

Mayonnaise (2 tablespoons) -

Butter (2 tablespoons)

- Chipotle peppers in adobo sauce (4 ounces) -

Garlic (2 cloves, pressed)

- Jalapeño (1 fresh, chopped) -

Olive oil (2 tablespoons)

- Yellow onion (half of an onion, diced)

What to do:

1. Fry diced onion (until translucent) in olive oil in a high sided pan, over medium- high heat.

2. Reduce heat to medium, add jalapeno and garlic. Cook while stirring for another two minutes.

3. Chop the chipotle peppers and add them, along with the adobo sauce, to the pan.

4. Add the butter, mayo, and fish fillets to the pan.

5. Cook the fish fully while breaking up the fillets and stirring the fish into other ingredients.

6. Warm tortillas for 2 minutes on each side.

7. Fill tortillas with fishy goodness and eat up!

3. SALMON WITH AVOCADO LIME SAUCE

Net Carbs: 5 grams

Protein: 37 grams

Fat: 27 grams

It takes 20 minutes to prepare, 10 minutes to cook, and serves
2. What you will need:

- Salmon (two 6 ounce fillets) -

Avocado (1 large)

- Lime (one-half of a whole lime) -

Red onion (2 tablespoons, diced) -

Cauliflower (100 grams)

What to do:

1. Chop cauliflower in a blender or food processor then cooks it in a lightly oiled pan, while covered, for 8 minutes. This will make the cauliflower rice-like.

2. Next, blend the avocado with squeezed lime juice in the blender or processor until smooth and creamy.

3. Heat some oil in a skillet and cook salmon (skin side down first) for 4 to 5 minute. Flip the fillets and cook for an additional 4 to 5 minutes.

4. Place salmon fillet on a bed of your cauliflower rice and top with some diced red onion.

4. SIRACHA LIME STEAK

Net Carbs: 5 grams

Protein: 48 grams

Fat: 32 grams

It takes 5 minutes to prepare, 10 minutes to cook, and serves 2.

What you will need:

- Vinegar (1 teaspoon)

- Olive oil (2 tablespoons) -

Lime (1 whole)

- Sriracha (2 tablespoons) -

Flank steak (16 ounces) -

Salt and pepper

What to do:

1. Season steak, liberally, with salt and pepper. Place on baking sheet, lined with foil, and broil in oven for 5 minutes on each side (add another minute or two for a well-done steak). Remove from oven, cover, and set aside.

2. Place sriracha in a small bowl and squeeze lime into it. Whisk in salt, pepper, and vinegar.

3. Slowly pour in olive oil.

4. Slice steak into thin slices, slather on your sauce, and enjoy!

5. Feel free to pair this recipe with a side of greens such as asparagus or broccoli.

5. LOW CARB SESAME CHICKEN

Net Carbs: 4 grams

Protein: 45 grams

Fat: 36 grams

Takes 15minutes to prepare, 15 minutes to cook, and serves

2. What you will need:

- Broccoli (three-fourths of a cup, cut bite size) -

Xanthan gum (a fourth of a teaspoon)

- Sesame seeds (2 tablespoons) -

Garlic (1 clove)

- Ginger (1 cm cube)

- Vinegar (1 tablespoon)

- Brown sugar alternative (Sukrin Gold is a good one) (2 tablespoons) -

Soy sauce (2 tablespoons)

- Toasted sesame seed oil (2 tablespoons)

- Arrowroot powder or cornstarch (1 tablespoon) -

Chicken thighs (1poundcut into bite sized pieces) -

Egg (1 large)

- Salt and pepper -

Chives (optional)

What to do:

1. First, we will make the batter by combining the egg with a tablespoon of arrowroot powder (or cornstarch). Whisk well.

2. Place chicken pieces in batter. Be sure to coat all sides of chicken pieces with the batter.

3. Heat one tablespoon of sesame oil, in a large pan. Add chicken pieces to hot oil and fry. Be gentle when flipping the chicken, you want to keep the batter from falling off. It should take about 10 minutes for them to cook fully.

4. Next, make the sesame sauce. In a small bowl, combine soy sauce, brown sugar alternative, vinegar, ginger, garlic, sesame seeds, and the remaining tablespoon of toasted sesame seed oil. Whisk very well.

5. Once the chicken is fully cooked, add broccoli and the sesame sauce to the pan and cook for an additional 5 minutes.

6. Spoon desired amount into a bowl, top it off with some chopped chives, and relish in some fine dining at home!

6. PAN 'O SAUSAGE

Net Carbs: 4 grams

Protein: 30 grams

Fat: 38 grams

It takes 10 minutes to prepare, 25 minutes to cook, and serves

2. What you will need:

- Basil (half a teaspoon)
- Oregano (half a teaspoon) -

White onion (1 tablespoon)

- Shredded mozzarella (a fourth of a cup) -

Parmesan cheese (a fourth of a cup)

- Vodka sauce (half a cup) -

Mushrooms (4 ounces) -

Sausage (3 links)

- Salt (a fourth of a teaspoon)
- Red pepper (a fourth of a teaspoon, ground)

What to do:

1. Preheat oven to 350 degrees Fahrenheit.

2. Heat an iron skillet over medium flame. When skillet is hot, cook sausage links until almost thoroughly cooked.

3. While sausage is cooking, slice mushrooms and onion.

4. When sausage is almost fully cooked, remove links from heat and place mushrooms and onions in skillet until brown.

5. Cut sausage into pieces about ½ inch thick and place pieces in the pan.

6. Season skillet contents with oregano, basil, salt, and red pepper.

7. Add vodka sauce and parmesan cheese. Stir everything together.

8. Place skillet in oven for 15 minutes. Sprinkle mozzarella on top a couple minutes before removing the dish from oven.

9. Once 15 minutes is up, remove skillet from the oven and let cool for a few minutes.

10. Dinner time!

7. QUARTER POUNDER KETO BURGER

Net Carbs: 4 grams

Protein: 25 grams

Fat: 34 grams

Takes 10 minutes to prepare, 8 minutes to cook, and serves

2. What you will need:

- Basil (half a teaspoon)

- Cayenne (fourth a teaspoon)

- Crushed red pepper (half a teaspoon)

- Salt (half a teaspoon)

- Lettuce (2 large leaves)

- Butter (2 tablespoons)

- Egg (1 large)

- Sriracha (1 tablespoon)

- Onion (fourth of whole onion)

- Plum tomato (half of the whole tomato)

- Mayo (1 tablespoon)

- Pickled jalapenos (1 tablespoon, sliced)

- Bacon (1 strip)

- Ground beef (half a pound)

- Bacon (1 strip)

What to do:

1. Knead mean for about three minutes.

2. Chop bacon, jalapeno, tomato, and onion into fine pieces. (shown below)

3. Knead in mayo, sriracha, egg, and chopped ingredients, and spices into the meat.

4. Separate meat into four even pieces and flatten them (not thinly, just press on the tops to create a flat surface). Place a tablespoon of butter on top of two of the meat pieces. Take the pieces that do not have butter in them and set them on top of the buttered ones (basically creating a butter and meat sandwich). Seal the sides together, concealing the butter within.

5. Throw the patties on the grill (or in a pan) for about 5 minutes on each side. Caramelize some onions if you want too!

6. Prepare large leaves of lettuce by spreading some mayo onto them. Once patties are finished, place them on one-half of the lettuce, add your desired burger toppings, and fold the other half over of the lettuce leaf over the patty.

7. Burger time!

...

...

BREAKFAST

Breakfast Recipes To Start Your Day Strong

Sconey Sconey Sunday – 6 SmartPoints Per Serving

This breakfast dish is best made on the weekend and enjoyed all week long. This breakfast should be filling in the moment due to the fluffiness of the scone and should keep you satisfied all morning because of the liberal use of peaches. If you are new to baking, or just a little bit afraid of your own oven, this is a great recipe to start with. There is no need to wait for any ingredients to rise and it builds the foundation for many other scone recipes. You can replace the peach with blueberries, banana, apple, etc. Try and experiment to find what you like most. Ready in 25 Minutes

10 minutes to prep and 15 minutes to cook

Ingredients (serves 4):

2/3 cups of all purpose flour

½ teaspoon of baking powder

½ teaspoon of baking soda

1 teaspoon of powdered sugar

2 tablespoons of sugar

½ teaspoon of half and half

1 teaspoon of margarine

1/3 cup of vanilla yogurt (I highly recommend Stoneyfield for the best results)

1 teaspoon of salt

3 tablespoons of chopped peaches (if you are using canned peaches, make sure you drain the peaches and give the peaches some time to dry. I recommend not using

128

canned as they tend to contain additional sugars that add unnecessary calories and distort the flavor of the peaches)

Non-stick cooking spray

Step 1:

Preheat the oven to 400 degrees F or 205 degrees

C Step 2:

Take a medium size mixing bowl and add the flour, sugar (not powdered), baking powder, baking soda, and salt. Mix the ingredients and add in the margarine while doing so. The margarine can be difficult to work with so you may want to heat it up in a microwave for 15 seconds, or alternatively cut the margarine into small pieces. Only move onto step 4 when you have a consistent base in the bowl – the margarine should be fully mixed in.

Step 3:

Add the yogurt and the peaches, mixing while you do so.

Step 4:

Take a large piece of wax paper and empty the contents of the bowl onto the paper. Knead the dough for 3-4 minutes. Many are unsure of how to knead the dough, so think about it as folding the dough over itself over and over.

Step 5:

Coat a large baking tray with non-stick spray and form the scones on the tray. The scones look best when shaped like triangles. The exact size of the scones is not as important as making sure the scones are of equal size. This recipe usually yields between 4 and 6 scones. Make sure the dough is firmly pressed against the baking tray. Bake for 12-15 minutes on the center oven rack. Step 6:

Remove the scones from the oven and while still hot, paint the scones with milk. This should look like they are slightly moist from the milk. Use this moisture to spread the powdered sugar over the scones. You can serve these right away and they will last about one week at room temperature.

10 Minute Fried Toast – 3 SmartPoints Per Serving

Yes this recipe is truly just a variation of French Toast but I want to stress the importance of a hot breakfast and that it doesn't take too much time to prepare one. This dish can be enjoyed even on a weekday before work and with a little practice you can cut down on the prep time dramatically. This is a dish I commonly make for my daughter before school and it can be made almost as fast as some simple scrambled eggs.

Ready in 10 Minutes

5 minutes to prep and 5 minutes to cook

Ingredients (serves 2):

4 egg whites

6 slices of wheat bread (you'll have lots of options of bread but I suggest looking at the low calorie version. I have switched to 40-45 calorie bread per slice and haven't noticed a big difference. The slices are a little smaller but each piece is less than half the calories of traditional white bread)

¼ cup of 1% milk

2 tablespoons of sugar free maple syrup (this recipe changes to 5 SmartPoints per serving with regular syrup)

1 tablespoon of cinnamon

1 tablespoon of vanilla extract

Non-stick cooking spray

Step 1:

In a shallow mixing bowl, add the egg whites, milk, and vanilla extract. Whisk these ingredients together.

Step 2:

Coat a skillet with cooking spray and put it over low-medium heat. Dip both sides of your wheat bread into the mixing bowl from step 1 and add to the skillet. You should be able to cook roughly 2 pieces at a time. Step 3:

While still hot, sprinkle cinnamon on each piece of toast. Serve with syrup and enjoy right away.

3 Minute Breakfast Mug – 2 SmartPoints Per Serving

Perhaps you thought 10 minutes was too long to dedicate to cooking a warm breakfast, well then this recipe is for you. This is a breakfast I used to make at the office as the ingredients can be stored easily in a refrigerator. You will absolutely need to use the liquid egg substitute as opposed to liquid eggs as the substitute will cook better in the microwave. If you have never used your microwave as a primary cooking tool, do not fear – this too was my first recipe cooked entirely in a microwave. When you get a look at the finished product you will be highly satisfied with the result – it tastes great too.

Ready in 3 Minutes

1 minute to prep and 2 minutes to cook

Ingredients (serves 1):

½ cup of liquid egg substitute

1 ounce of low-fat turkey breast (optional)

1 slice of American cheese

Non-stick cooking spray

Step 1:

Take a microwave-safe mug and coat it with the non-stick spray.

Step 2:

Pour the egg substitute into the mug and microwave on high for 1 minute.

Step 3:

Add in the cheese and optionally the turkey. If you're adding the turkey, you will want to make sure that it is in very fine pieces. Microwave for an additional minute.

Saturday Morning Enriching Oatmeal – 7 SmartPoints

This filling breakfast will have you thinking differently about oatmeal. We take a hearty essential oatmeal recipe and add a combination of zesty flavors that make the dish shine. This breakfast takes longer than the others to cook and is best enjoyed on a weekend, or when you have some extra time before starting your day. This recipe can easily be doubled or tripled to serve the entire family. Ready in 30 Minutes

10 minutes to prep and 20 minutes to cook

Ingredients (serves 1):

½ cup raw oats

2 teaspoons of lemon juice

1/8 teaspoon of cinnamon

1/8 teaspoon of salt

1 low-calorie sweetener packet similar to Splenda

1 cup of unsweetened almond milk, or vanilla soy milk

1 cup of water

Step 1:

In a small pot, combine the oats, cinnamon, salt, almond milk, and water.

Step 2:

Heat the pot on high heat and bring the oatmeal to a near boil. Once bubbling reduce the heat to low. Cook for 10-15 minutes after the oatmeal has been put to low heat.

Step 3:

Stir occasionally and remove from burner when the oatmeal has thickened.

Step 4:

Before serving, add the sweetener packet to the serving bowl.

Lunch Recipes That Will Keep You Satisfied All Afternoon

Home Joe's Mediterranean Hummus With Pita Bread – 4 Smart Points Per Serving

This recipe is based on a small love affair I have for the Trader Joe's Mediterranean Hummus. I have tweaked this recipe to get very much the same taste, but with all the added benefit of knowing exactly what ingredients are used. This hummus is packed full of healthy fats from the chick peas, fats that will leave you satisfied all afternoon. I love to bring a small container to work and pair it with either pita chips or pita bread and a side of fresh vegetables – carrots and peppers in particular. Be on the lookout for the nutritional information on the chips or pita bread of your choice – while the hummus is healthy, aim for a serving of less than 200 calories for whatever you choose to dip in the hummus and add 2 smart points to the meal. Feel free to use as many veggies as you want for dipping though, think about these as 0 points.

Ready in 30 Minutes

30 minutes to prepare.

Ingredients (serves 8):

A food processor that can hold 3 cups

1 large garlic glove

2 tablespoons of tahini

½ lemon

6 tablespoons of extra virgin olive oil (the taste is important here, so use extra virgin instead of "pure")

¼ teaspoon of cumin

1 teaspoon of crushed red pepper

½ cup of boiling water

Step 0:

This recipe is dependent on your food processor. You won't need to prepare any ingredients, but make sure that your processor is up to the task. I have had this recipe come out just a tad too lumpy in the past because of the food processor, so blending time may vary slightly to get the consistency that you want. Step 1:

Put the garlic clove and the processor and pulse 3 to 4 times. Add the rest of the ingredients except for the water.

Step 2:

Run the processor for 3-5 minutes, periodically switching from pulse to long sustained processing.

Step 3:

Pour in the hot water (does not need to be exactly boiling) and run the processor for an additional 30 seconds to a minute. Check the consistency of the hummus and run the processor for additional time if needed. You may need to add more than ½ a cup of water depending in the consistency of the beans and how powerful your food processor is.

Step 4:

With the desired consistency, pour the hummus in to a container and store in the fridge for several hours. Serving right away will not yield the best flavor as the ingredients are still settling.

Step 5 (Optional):

If serving for a party or if you simply want slightly more indulgent hummus, add a drizzle of olive oil to the hummus before serving.

5 Minute Turkey Wrap – 8 SmartPoints Per Serving

I ate these wraps nearly three times a week for half a year – they were just that delicious. They're easy to make and great to bring as a bagged lunch. Ready in 5 Minutes

5 minutes to prep and 0 minutes to cook

Ingredients (serves 1)

3 ounces of low-sodium turkey breast (I encourage you to use your local deli counter versus the prepackaged meats – the deli counter meats will often have less sodium so even if you aren't purchasing 'low-sodium' turkey, it is probably still worth it to buy from the deli counter)

1 ounce of lettuce or spinach

¼ of one whole tomato

1 tablespoon of low-fat ranch dressing

1 ounce of low-fat mozzarella cheese (you can use other cheeses, but for the calorie to size ratio, I find mozzarella to be the best investment)

1 wrap or flatbread that is between 100-150 calories per wrap/flatbread (your supermarket will have several options for you but I suggest the Flatout Wraps. These wraps are fluffy and delicious are only 90 calories. For wraps above 150 calories, add another SmartPoint to the recipe)

Step 1:

Take out your wrap or flatbread and heat it in the microwave for 15-20 seconds – this will fluff up your wrap and make it more malleable to shape. Step 2:

Spread your low-fat ranch dressing over the wrap. Fill the wrap with your turkey, lettuce or spinach, tomatoes, and cheese. Step 3:

Roll up your wrap and store for lunch or eat right away.

Slow Cooker Southern Style Chicken Soup -4 SmartPoints Per Serving

It's an all day affair that that will last you all week and then some. This hearty soup is great in the winter and full of exotic blends of flavors that will have you wondering why you don't eat soup more often. Since this recipe produces a fairly large batch, it's worth noting that this soup freezes extremely well. If you decide to freeze individual servings, simply let the soup thaw at room temperature before you reheat in the microwave – this is the best way to preserve the flavor. Ready in 7 Hours

10 minutes to prep and 6-8 hours to cook

Ingredients (serves 10)

2 large chicken breasts cut into inch size cubes

1 clove of finely minced garlic

1 cup of corn (canned is what I use)

½ diced large white onion

½ cup of finely chopped chilantro

1 teaspoon of cumin

1 tablespoon of chili powder

15 ounces of washed and drained kidney beans (canned is what I use)

15 ounces of washed and drained black beans (canned is what I use)

1 teaspoon of lime juice

2 whole bell peppers cut into long strips

1 15 ounce can of diced tomatoes

Pepper to taste

Salt to taste

Step 1:

Prepare all of your ingredients and pour them into your slow cooker. Put the slow cookers on low heat and let cook for 6-8 hours. To make sure that the soup is done, reach for a piece of chicken and slice to find the color in the center. Note that it is very difficult to overcook this recipe – even 9 hours in the slow cooker will result in a fantastic soup.

Alternative: If you do not have a slow cooker, do not fret – a regular pot on low heat on your burner will do just fine. There are some limitations however in that you will need to be present the entire time the soup is cooking. It is also possible to overcook the soup if you are using a traditional pot (I first made this recipe using this method and it turned out great. It does require time and patience if you're using a pot, but it can be made over the weekend and enjoyed all week long).

Healthy Zone Calzone – 4 SmartPoints Per Serving

I love this recipe because it uses a neat trick – we substitute heavy dough for Pillsbury and get to cut down on the cooking time in the process. This dish is great by itself and works great as a lunch served at room temperature. If you decide to make the marinara sauce in the next chapter, try it as a dipping sauce for this delicious healthy calzone.

Ready in 40 Minutes

25 minutes to prep and 15 minutes to cook

Ingredients (serves 8):

1 can of reduced fat crescent rolls by Pillsbury (this is absolutely necessary to get the right amount of dough to calorie ratio)

¼ cup of reduce fat shredded cheese (mozzarella is my go to choice but feel free to use your favorite).

6 ounces of low-fat chicken breast

2 cups of baby spinach

6 tablespoons of low-fat whipped cream cheese (you can also use reduced fat but know that it changes the total SmartPoints per serving quite significantly).

1-2 tablespoons of vegetable oil

Step 1:

Take the chicken breast and cut it into cubes before cooking in a frying pan. Use the vegetable oil to cook the chicken and try to use the least amount of oil possible. This recipe is extremely lean and the vegetable oil is actually one of the more calorie expensive ingredients – any savings here do add up. Step 2:

Preheat the oven to 375 degrees F or 190 degrees C.

Step 3:

Remove the Pillsbury rolls and arrange them on an ungreased baking tray. The container should contain 8 rolls but we are only making 4 calzones. Combine rolls to make the 4 calzones and make sure each roll is flat on the tray. Step 4:

Spread over each roll the baby spinach, cream cheese, chicken, and your choice of shredded cheese. These rolls are fairly small for how stuffed these calzones will be (definitely a good thing), so you may need to kneed some of the ingredients into the dough itself – this works particularly well with the cream cheese and shredded cheese.

Step 5:

Form each of the individual 4 calzones, fold the dough over the ingredients and 'close' the calzone. This step can be a little tricky if the dough is not at room temperature. The final shape should look a little bit like a crescent moon

Step 6:

Bake for 10-15 minutes in the middle rack of the oven. You will know when the calzones are ready as the dough will begin to flake and turn brown.

8 Minute Tuna – 3 SmartPoints Per Serving

I still prepare this Tuna Salad at least twice a month. It's quick and easy and great to bring to work. If you feel like you're missing out on the pure indulgence of 'fatty' flavors then this salad will hit the spot. Even though we are using low-fat mayonnaise, it still hits all the right notes and you'd be hard pressed to tell the difference between this and a much more calorie dense mayonnaise base. One of the greatest aspects of this recipe, and why it's only 3 SmartPoints per serving, is the use of lettuce as the base for wraps.

We use lettuce for a couple of reasons: one, the neutral flavor of the lettuce brings out the creaminess of the salad without distorting the taste and two, the crispness of the lettuce is essential for the proper texture. I came up with the idea for using lettuce as a base after eating Korean barbeque. Try it and you'll see how it really does bring out the flavor.

Ready in 8 Minutes

8 minutes to prep and 0 minutes to cook

Ingredients (serves 4):

12 ounces of albacore white tuna in water (essential as this tuna has the meatiest texture and taste)

3 tablespoons of low-fat mayonnaise

3 stalks o chopped celery (if any part of the stalk is not hard, then do not use that section. You want the celery to be firm as to add a crunchiness to the salad).

1 teaspoon of Dijon mustard

½ teaspoon of black pepper

½ teaspoon of table-salt (do not use sea-salt as the harsher grain does not spread as evenly throughout the salad)

½ head of lettuce cut into large pieces (these will serve as the wraps for eating the tuna so keep that in mind as you cut the lettuce)

Step 1:

Drain the tuna and add to a large mixing bowl. Add the celery, pepper, salt, mustard, and mayonnaise. Stir well, breaking up the large pieces of tuna that might be sticking together from the can.

Step 2:

For best results, leave the salad in the fridge for 20 minutes to let thicken.

Serve with the large pieces of lettuce.

Week-Long Rice With Chicken – 4 SmartPoints Per Serving

One of the essentials of preparing a good lunch is not having to worry about side dishes. This dish comes with everything you need – protein to keep you full, carbohydrates to give you afternoon energy, and veggies for your general nutrition and to flavor the dish. This rice dish can be stored away for work and can be enjoyed at room temperature or even cold – it will still taste delicious! Ready in 30 Minutes

15 minutes to prep and 15 minutes to cook

Ingredients (serves 6):

2 large lean, boneless chicken breasts

2 large eggs

2 cups uncooked brown rice

½ cup of pea

½ cup of chopped carrots

2 finely chopped cloves of garlic

2 tablespoons of soy sauce (1 tablespoon if using low-sodium soy sauce – better results are gotten with regular soy)

4 tablespoons of water

Non-stick cooking spray or if unavailable, 1 tablespoon of vegetable oil

Step 1:

Take the chicken breast and cut the chicken into long strips. The important part of cutting the chicken is that each strip has roughly the same thickness. Do not worry about how thick or thin your chicken is – just make sure it is fairy uniform. Step 2:

Cook the brown rice on your stovetop. Use 5 cups of water for the 2 cups of brown rice. This is more water than is typically used and you will need to cook the rice for slightly longer. The rice will fluff up much more with that extra cup of water. Move onto step 3 only after the rice is done. Step 3:

In a large skillet, scramble the two large eggs and set aside.

Step 4:

Coat the same skillet again with non-stick cooking spray. Each skillet is a little bit difference and if you know that non-stick spray is not going to be able to grease the entire pan, use 1 tablespoon of vegetable oil, as we do not want the chicken to stick to the pan. Add the sliced chicken and cook halfway before adding the carrots. As the chicken starts to look fully cooked, add the chopped garlic and peas.

Step 4:

Take the soy sauce and pour it into a small dish with the water. Mix and pour into the skillet. The water will evaporate and ensure that the soy sauce is not too overpowering. Move onto step 5 once the chicken is fully cooked and the water is mostly evaporated.

Step 5:

Add into the skillet the cooked rice and scrambled eggs. Mix well and remove from the burner once the eggs have warmed up. Serve right away.

Admiral David's Broccoli – 5 SmartPoints Per Serving

If the name seems familiar, or just a bit off, that's because it is indeed a variation of General Tso's Chicken. It's a standard American Chinese dish that incorporates crisp chicken, spice, and a tinge of orange flavoring. This recipe is derived from a dish a college roommate of mine used to make. If you guessed his name is David, then you would be correct. As with many of the other lunch dishes, this one is also great when served cold. This dish is a complete meal and doubles as a fantastic dinner that is quick to make.

Ready in 25 Minutes

15 minutes to prep and 10 minutes to cook

Ingredients (serves 4):

2 large chicken breasts

1 orange, cut and peeled

1 teaspoon of corn starch

4 teaspoon of vegetable oil

1 bag of precut broccoli florets (should equal roughly 2 cups)

1 tablespoon of minced ginger

¼ cup water (to mix with soy

sauce) 3 tablespoons of soy sauce

¼ cup of orange juice

½ cup of chicken or vegetable broth

½ cup water (for help in cooking broccoli)

Step 1:

Take the chicken breasts and cut into long strips. Add the soy sauce to the ¼ cup of water and mix, set aside. During this step, make sure that your other ingredients are all set and ready to go. Once the pan heats up the cooking processes is very fast.

Step 2:

Add the vegetable oil to a large skillet warm over medium heat. Add the chicken strips and cook halfway – add the ginger and continue to cook the chicken until it is entirely done. Take the chicken and ginger out of the skillet and set aside. Step 3:

Return to the skillet and add the broccoli. You should not need to add any additional oil but if when removing the chicken the pan was left dry, add an additional teaspoon. As the broccoli starts to lightly brown add the ½ cup of water and cover the skillet. Let the broccoli steam for 3 minutes. Check the broccoli to make sure that it is cooked through and not too raw. Step 4:

Add the cooked chicken and ginger to the skillet. Add the soy sauce mixed with water, the orange juice, and the chicken broth. Mix these ingredients well and allow to cook for an additional 5 minutes. If the chicken or broccoli is beginning to be overcooked, change the heat to low or turn off the burner. Step 5:

Add in the cornstarch and continue to mix. Once the cornstarch has been mixed in, add the orange peels to the top of the dish and cook for an additional minute or two. Serve right away.

Dinner Recipes For The Healthy Body

Lightning Fast Curry Noodles – 3 SmartPoints Per Serving

This is a recipe I commonly refer to when I'm looking to make a quick dinner with just a bit of Asian flair. My favorite aspect to this recipe is that by using rice noodles you do not need to cook the noodles in a pot of boiling water. It can be made with just about any protein, including eggs or tofu. This particular version is vegetarian free, but adding cooked chicken or beef works just as well. This is my own recipe is supposed to mimic Singapore Noodles, a dish commonly found at Chinese restaurants throughout the country. Ready In 20 Minutes:

10 minutes to prepare and 10 minutes to cook Ingredients (serves 4)

3 large eggs

2 tablespoons whole milk (or half and half)

3 teaspoons of curry powder

2 tablespoons of vegetable oil

2 whole white mushrooms

1 bell pepper

1 package of Rice Noodles (you will want to go for medium thickness in the noodle – the particular brand does not matter)

2 tablespoons of soy sauce (low sodium soy sauce will *taste* more salty than regular soy sauce. If using low sodium soy then only use 1 tablespoon)

Step 1:

Take a large bowl or pot and fill it with warm water. The water does not need to approach boiling, and running hot water from your tap will suffice. Once the bowl is full, put the package of rice noodles into the water. You want to check back in a few minutes to make sure that every noodle is submerged in the water. Step 2: Slice the mushrooms and bell peppers into small slices. This dish will look a lot like a noodle stir fry, so cut the peppers in long strips and the mushrooms into thin slices.

Step 3:

While the noodles are soaking, use a small frying pan and with the milk and 3 eggs, make scrambled eggs. Once the eggs are made put them aside on a separate plate and cut the scrambled eggs into small pieces.

Step 4:

As the eggs are cooking, take a pan suitable for stir fry and add the vegetable oil. If you do not have a suitable stir fry pan, you can also use a standard pot for boiling pasta. Bring the heat to medium high and once the oil is hot add the mushrooms. As the mushrooms start to cook, add the peppers.

Step 5:

Strain the rice and noodles and add them to the pan with the mushrooms and the bell peppers. Note that the noodles should still appear to be a little bit brittle, do not worry as they will continue to cook in the pan. Step 6:

As the noodles are cooking in the pan, add the soy sauce and mix thoroughly. Once the sauce is mixed, add the curry powder and stir thoroughly. The noodles should start to take on a dark yellowish color and at this point they should be thoroughly cooked through.

Step 7:

Add the cooked eggs to the pan, and then serve immediately. If the scrambled eggs are slightly cold, they will be warmed up through the cooked noodles. Step 8:

Serve immediately and enjoy! This meal also works great for lunch. If you are unable to reheat the noodles while at work, they taste great just at room temperature.

Simple Season Chicken– 3 SmartPoints Per Serving

This recipe is a great healthy way to make seasoned chicken cutlets. These cutlets have just the right amount of seasoning and come packed with all the healthy protein of lean chicken breast. This recipe can altered slightly to make a lean type of chicken parmesan. See the altered steps 4 and 5 if you wish to go this route, otherwise this recipe is great with a side of spinach or any other side vegetable.

Ready In 35 Minutes

10 minutes to prepare and 25 minutes to cook

Ingredients (serves 4)

Chicken breast (use roughly 1 pound and cut into 4 large filets)

1/8 teaspoon paprika

¼ cup of parmesan cheese (grated

finely) ½ teaspoon of garlic powder

1 teaspoon of parsley (optional)

black pepper to taste

3 tablespoons of dried

breadcrumbs Directions:

Step 1:

Preheat your oven to 400 degrees F or 205 degrees

C Step 2:

Take a small mixing bowl and add the breadcrumbs, grated parmesan, garlic powder, and paprika. Add a pinch of black pepper but know that you can add more while the chicken is cooking.

Step 3:

Take your sliced pieces of chicken breast and dip them into the bowl. Coat both sides of each piece of chicken. Since we are using a healthier version of traditional chicken parmesan, you might have some difficult having the mix stick to the chicken. It is best dip the chicken in the bowl right after you wash the chicken, using the moisture to get it to stick properly.

Step 4:

Prepare a nonstick baking tray and align the pieces of chicken towards the center of the baking tray.

Alternate for Chicken Parmesan: Using the Homemade Multi-Purpose Marina sauce (the next recipe in the book), lather the chicken liberally in 2-3 cups of sauce. You will need to use a deeper baking dish to cook the Chicken Parmesan. Once the sauce and chicken has been laid out, coat with shredded Parmesan Cheese and whole slices of mozzarella. To use an appropriate amount of cheese, only layer the cheese on top of the chicken filets. Note that this adds roughly 2 Smart Points to each serving.

Step 5:

Let the chicken bake in the oven for 25 minutes. Check at about 20 minutes as thinner pieces of chicken will cook more quickly. 25 minutes is around the upper limit for how long it will take to cook the chicken.

Alternate for Chicken Parmesan: Using the oven set to 400 degrees F, bake for 35-40 minutes.

Step 6: Remove the chicken form the baking tray and serve within 5-10 minutes.

Homemade Multi-Purpose Marinara – 3 Smart Points Per Serving

This is a great recipe to try out on the weekend and use all week long. Whether it's topping for Chicken Parmesan, dipping sauce for bread, or the foundation of a great pasta dish, this marinara sauce will leave you with plenty of options for how to enjoy it.

Ready in 30 Minutes

10 minutes to prepare and 20 minutes to cook Ingredients (makes 1 quart)

2 large cloves of garlic

4 large tomatoes

1 28 ounce can of peeled tomatoes

3 tablespoons of olive oil (use extra virgin olive oil – the taste will make a huge difference)

1 ½ tablespoons of sugar

½ teaspoon of ground black pepper 1 teaspoon of salt

½ large white onion

Step 1:

Take your fresh tomatoes and dice them into small chunks. You can also optionally peel the skin from the tomatoes for a smoother sauce. During this step also chop your half onion and your garlic cloves.

Step 2:

In large sauce pan, heat the olive oil under a medium heat, add the diced onion. Wait until the onion is firmly sautéing before adding the garlic.

Step 3:

Add your chopped tomatoes and your can of tomatoes. Also stir in your black pepper and salt. Bring the heat up to medium high and wait for the sauce to boil. Stir frequently and let the sauce boil for 15 minutes. Step 4:

Turn the heat down to low on the burner and let the sauce simmer for an additional 30 minutes.

Savory Grilled Salmon – 4 Smart Points Per Serving

If there's a common theme with this cookbook, it's the idea that healthy proteins are the foundation to a great diet. Even if you do not normally love salmon, or if you've never tried it, this recipe is certainly worth a shot. At 4 SmartPoints per serving, a side dish of potatoes and spinach will bring the total meal to a reasonable 6-7 SmartPoints, meanwhile the salmon will keep you full until morning. Ready in 50 Minutes

30 minutes to prep and 20 minutes to cook

Ingredients (serves 4):

1 pound of skinless salmon fillet. You will want the thickness of the salmon to be about 1 inch.

¼ cup of soy sauce Non-

stick cooking spray

1 tablespoon of rice wine vinegar

¼ cup of dry sherry

1 tablespoon of brown sugar

1 teaspoon of garlic powder

1/8 teaspoon of ginger

Black pepper to taste

Step 1:

Preheat the oven to 375 degrees F or 190 degrees C. Make sure the grill rack is in the center of the oven.

Step 2:

Combine the sherry, soy sauce, brown sugar, vinegar, garlic powder, and ginger in a mixing bowl.

Step 3:

Dip the filets of salmon in the mixing bowl and place in the refrigerator for 20 minutes to marinade.

Step 4:

Place the remaining marinade in a small saucepan and heat on low. The marinade will begin to thicken as the salmon marinades in the refrigerator. Step 5:

Spray the grill rack with non-stick spray and place the salmon filets on the rack. The cooking time for the salmon will differ greatly depending on thickness. As a guideline each side will need 4 to 8 minutes to cook through. The sign that the salmon is fully cooked is when it begins to flake. Step 6:

Remove the salmon from the oven and place it on a large serving plate. Coat the salmon in the remaining marinade. Serve immediately.

Cheesy Baked Chicken – 5 SmartPoints Per Serving

I love this dish if for no other reason than it remind me that dieting does not need to omit cream and cheese. This chicken dish has all the flavor of a delicious casserole without any of the guilt. A simple side dish like a lightly tossed salad goes great, just be sure not to overdo it with the dressing. Ready in 55 minutes:

10 minutes to prep and 45 minutes to cook

Ingredients (serves 8):

2 cups of cooked macaroni noodles

2 cups of 1% fat skin milk

2 cups of chopped boneless chicken breasts cut into cubes

8 ounces of low-fat shredded cheddar cheese

2 cups of undiluted cream of mushroom soup (I personally use Campbell's brand)

Step 1:

Preheat the oven to 350 degrees F or 175 degrees C.

Step 2:

Use a baking dish that is 2 inches deep, similar to a casserole dish, and place the cream of mushroom soup, the skim milk, cooked macaroni, shredded cheese, and uncooked chicken breasts into the baking tray. Mix thoroughly. Step 3:

Place the baking tray in the center oven rack and bake for 35 minutes. At 35 minutes, take the baking tray out of the oven and remove a piece of chicken. Cut the chicken in half to see if it is cooked all the way through. Typically this recipe calls for 45 minutes, but if the chicken pieces are small enough the dish could be done in 35. Cook for an additional 10 minutes if needed. Step 4:

45 minutes is the upper limit for cooking the casserole, but always make sure to slice the chicken and make sure that it is cooked all the way through. Small variables could mean cooking for an additional 5-10 minutes. Step 5:

Let the dish cook for 10 minutes before serving.

Lean Mean Pork Chops – 3 SmartPoints Per Serving

In this recipe we are using our oven to bypass the unnecessary oil we'd get in by using a frying pan. This will lead to a more brazen pork that should be more tender. This dish takes longer than several of our other dinners and so use this time to experiment with side dishes. A vegetable melody goes great as the extra time gives you the opportunity to wash and cut your vegetables. You can also use the already heated oven for simple sliced baked potatoes – even the spices from the pork can be reused if you wish.

Ready in 70 Minutes

20 minutes to prep and 50 minutes to cook

Ingredients Needed (serves 4):

Non-stick cooking spray

1 large egg white

¼ teaspoon of ground ginger

1/8 teaspoon of garlic powder

2 tablespoon of pineapple juice

6 ounces of pork loin (try and get lean pork if available)

1 tablespoon of soy sauce

¼ teaspoon of paprika

1/3 cup dried breadcrumbs

¼ teaspoon of dried Italian seasoning

Step 1:

Preheat the oven to 350 degrees F or 175 degrees

C Step 2:

If you were able to purchase lean pork loin then you do not need to follow this step. If you were not able to purchase lean pork loin, trim away as much fat as you can. Do not worry about the taste – our seasoning will make up for the flavor.

Step 3:

In large mixing bowl, add the soy sauce, garlic powder, egg white, ginger, and pineapple juice. Mix well as the egg white is sometimes difficult to mix thoroughly.

Step 4:

Using a separate bowl, mix breadcrumbs, Italian seasoning, and the paprika.

Step 5:

Take the pork chops and dip them into the wet mixing bowl and then dip them into the dry mixing bowl. Coat the pork chops well but know that some ingredients will be left.

Step 6:

Lay the pork chops on the baking tray. Bake for 25-30 minutes on each side.

Wait 3-5 minutes before serving.

Fast Cooking Scallops – 3 SmartPoints Per Serving

The hardest part of this recipe is the trip to the supermarket to purchase scallops. Do not fear as frozen scallops will work just fine, and if you are inexperienced cooking fish you also do not have to worry – this recipe is built upon the idea that perhaps this is your first time cooking fish in a pan. If you are unsure about whether to try this recipe, think about scallops as the 'meatier' shrimp. For a side dish, I recommend a baked potato and spinach or zucchini. The lemon goes great with subtle side dishes like these.

Ready in 20 Minutes

10 minutes to prep and 10 minutes to cook

Ingredients (serves 4):

1 pound of sea scallops, dried

2 tablespoons of all purpose flour

1 tablespoon of virgin olive oil

1 tablespoon of lemon juice

1 minced scallions

¼ teaspoon of salt

2 tablespoons of parsley

Pinch of sage (nice flavor, but not necessary if you don't already have this spice)

Step 1:

Take a mixing bowl and add the flour, scallions, and salt.

Step 2:

Take the scallops and dip them in the mixing bowl. Don't worry about how much of the mix ends up on the scallions – it should only be a small layer and does not necessary need to cover the scallops entirely. Step 3:

Take a large skillet and heat the olive oil under medium heat. Toss the scallops one at a time into the pan. The scallops should could in about 4 minutes. Be careful not to overcook the scallops as they will become very though. You will know the scallops are done when they become impossible to see through the skin.

Step 4:

If the scallops were made in batches, add all of the scallops back into the pan, turning off the heat before you do so. Add the chopped parsley and lemon juice. Mix well and serve right away.

PART 6

Chapter 1: What Is the DASH Effect?

Are you suffering from hypertension? Do you need a great way to lower your sodium intake without losing the flavor in your meals? If you are searching for the most successful diet plan, then this is your book. The DASH effect diet was ranked the best diet for 7 years in a row by the United States News and World Report. If you've been looking for a weight loss program, then the DASH effect is exactly what you need.

The DASH effect diet is a diet designed to help reduce hypertension and lower blood pressure by providing a diet of clean, fresh foods with lots of color variety. By lowering your sodium intake, you can lower your blood pressure. It's also known to lower your blood sugar which makes it great for diabetics. So what is the DASH effect? Well, DASH is an acronym for 'Dietary Approaches to Stop Hypertension.' With many Americans suffering from hypertension, having a healthy diet full of fresh, clean foods is something that everyone needs.

Since the DASH effect started, it has been making headlines. It is promoted by the National Heart, Lung and Blood Institute for hypertension and blood pressure. The USDA says that the DASH effect is the ideal plan for Americans, and the Kidney

Foundation has endorsed it for people suffering from kidney disease. With endorsements like these, why is everyone not following the DASH effect diet plan? The true answer is that change is hard. But the DASH effect diet doesn't have to be.

So what exactly is the DASH effect and how can you incorporate it into your life? Well, that is really quite easy. Since most of you are already eating the key foods in the DASH effect, it should not be much of a drastic change. I think the biggest change is the lower sodium intake. You see, in a normal American diet, we consume around 3,500mg of sodium per day. In the DASH effect diet plan, we want to lower our sodium intake. So why should we do that? Lowering our sodium intake to either 2,300mg per day or 1,500mg per day can make changes that will transform our health.

By lowering our sodium we can remedy our hypertension, also known as 'blood pressure,' and even reduce our systolic blood pressure. But that isn't all, we can also reduce blood sugar levels, and it aids in preventing osteoporosis, cancer, stroke, and diabetes. The added reward is by reducing our sodium intake and eating a cleaner more natural diet we are also reducing our caloric intake and thus by reducing our weight. Even though weight loss is not the reason for this dietary plan, it is an added benefit. Everyone is interested in losing weight and with the DASH effect diet you can do just that without missing out on caffeine, alcohol, sweets, fruits, vegetables, dairy, grains, or even dairy.

How do we do this? Well, it is as simple as portion control and choosing the proper ingredients for our meals. For instance, if you're having breakfast you would have:

> One store-bought, whole-wheat bagel with two tablespoons of peanut
> butter, without added salt of course
1 medium orange
One cup of low-fat milk or lactose-free milk
And 1 cup of decaffeinated coffee, without the sugar and cream

In the example above, not only do you have your wheat on your bagel, but you also have your protein in your peanut butter along with your coffee, dairy, and a fruit. Having this combination for breakfast will fill you up for the day while lowering your blood pressure. Each of these items is low in sodium, high in potassium, magnesium, and calcium. This breakfast gives you grains, fruit, dairy, and protein you'll need to start the day as recommended by the DASH effect diet meal plan. The best part about the DASH Effect is that you still get to have your caffeine, which helps boost your energy for the day ahead. This breakfast will provide you with the necessary nutrients that are needed to start your day on a healthy note.

The DASH effect is not like any other diet that you may have heard of. For instance, you do not have to eliminate your favorite foods. You just have to make a smarter choice when purchasing or preparing those foods. The DASH effect diet plan is so rich in potassium, magnesium, and calcium it provides a stronger foundation for your 2,000 calories nutritional intake that is recommended by the

USDA for the average person. If you need a higher calorie diet, you can increase the intake of vegetables, fruits, and proteins to build a healthier balanced diet and still follow the DASH effect program.

So, "What can I eat in the DASH effect plan?" you may be asking. Well, you might be surprised to find that you can eat almost everything you already eat. It's a cleaner dietary plan with many great meal prep options that we will discuss later in this book. The DASH effect diet plan offers items such as fresh, clean, low-fat, and not processed foods. For example, you can eat fruits, vegetables, low-fat dairy, whole grains, fish, poultry, and nuts. In limited quantities, you can have beef, sweets, and sugary beverages. Caffeine and alcohol are not included in this meal plan. However, you can follow the USDA recommendation of an intake of no more than 2 alcoholic or caffeinated beverages for males per day, and no more than 1 alcoholic or caffeinated beverage for women per day. With caffeine, it is best to switch to decaffeinated beverages and eliminate the sugar and heavy cream. However, if you do have sugar in your coffee or heavy cream, you want to deduct that from your permissible caloric intake per day.

So what exactly are your permissible servings per day with the DASH effect meal plan for each food item? Let's start with your grains. You are allowed 7-8 grains per day. One serving of grains is equivalent to one slice of bread or 0.50 cup of pasta or rice. This is based on a 2,000-calorie diet per day. If you need a higher calorie intake diet, then it is suggested you do not add more grains to your servings intake, instead add more fruit or vegetables.

Your allowable vegetable servings per day are 4-5 servings. Suggested vegetables range from broccoli, carrots, tomatoes, sweet potatoes, Brussels sprouts, and other greens. A serving size is one cup of raw salad greens or a 0.50 cup of chopped vegetables. Your vegetable intake can be cooked or raw. You can use frozen or fresh vegetables. You can also have stir fry or à la carte vegetables. Adding a few extra vegetables to your meals is recommended instead of adding sweets or grains.

Fruit is another recommended dietary choice. You can have 4-5 servings of fruit per day. These servings can consist of bananas, apples, grapes, berries, and more. A medium sized fruit or 0.50 cup of fresh or frozen fruit is the suggested serving size. Fruits are a great way to have a light snack throughout the day. They also provide necessary natural sugars to your diet. Just make sure you follow the serving suggestions for snacks and meals.

Dairy is something we all struggle with. We either can't stomach it, or we drink too much heavy creams and whole milk. On the DASH effect diet plan, we can have low-fat or fat-free dairy products. These can be milk, yogurt, cheese, and other dairy items. We should have no more than 2-3 servings of dairy per day. Lactose-free products are listed within this category as well. Each serving size should be no more than one cup of milk or yogurt per serving.

If you choose to incorporate meat into your DASH food prep, then consider that you should have no more than six servings of meat per day. Each serving is 1 ounce. In most diets, we should only eat about two 3-ounce servings of meat a week. A standard deck of cards or the area of the palm of your hand is about 3 ounces of meat. It is best to have only grilled, baked, or broiled meats. Your meat choices should consist of lean ground beef, salmon, turkey, tuna, and chicken. Tuna and salmon are high in omega-3 fatty acids and helps lower cholesterol. Meat is not a required item for the DASH effect diet, so whether you add meat or not is a choice you will have to make.

Supplementing meat with legumes is perfectly fine as well. Legumes fall in the seeds category and no more than 4-5 servings per day should be consumed. These are almonds, sunflower seeds, kidney beans, peas, lentils, and other beans and nut seeds that are high in omega-3 fatty acids and monounsaturated fat. They are great to sprinkle on salads, stir-fry, and add a nice crunch to any meal. One nut to stay away from is coconuts, they do not provide the proper nutrients that you would need for this plan. A serving size for legumes is two tablespoons of sunflower seeds or 0.33 cup of nuts or beans.

You are allowed at least 2-3 servings of fats and oils per day on the DASH effect diet plan. Oils such as olive oil, margarine, and low-fat mayonnaise are all allowable oils for condiments and adding flavor. One serving size is one tablespoon of soft margarine or mayonnaise.

Although we should all avoid sweets and sugar since they add fat to our bodies, on the DASH effect diet plan there is room for five or fewer servings of sweets per week. Allowable sugars are jelly, sorbet, hard candies, and more. A serving size is one tablespoon of sugar or 0.50 cup sorbet. When adding these in try to find low-fat or fat-free options. Even low-fat cookies are a great option for you, just remember to keep track of any other ingredients that were added to the cookies like nuts.

If you are like most people, you start your day with a cup of coffee with cream and sugar. Even though these things can cause the inflammation of your body, they are allowed in the DASH effect diet plan. Men should not have more than 2 drinks per day of either coffee or alcohol, and women should have no more than 1 drink of coffee or alcohol. This is another great advantage to this dietary plan. So if you are a heavy coffee drinker, or if you love that glass of wine at night before bed, this is where the struggle might come in. By limiting the intake of these drinks, we will feel healthier, and our blood sugar will be lowered drastically as well as limit the inflammatory effects of caffeine on our body.

Why does it work?

Through extensive research and open trials conducted by the National Institute of Health, the data collected showed the patients with hypertension, high blood pressure, and diabetes experienced a decrease of symptoms while they were on the DASH effect diet plan. By gradually changing your eating habits to follow the

DASH effect diet plan you are reducing your sodium intake and allowing your body to start healing. Start with one day a week and gradually work to a full week of eating healthy.

By changing your meal prep and choices for each meal, including snacks, you can gradually move up a day until you have fully integrated the DASH effect plan for every meal, seven days a week. Eliminate the sodium by not adding any more sodium to your meal prep and using an option for your foods that have a lower sodium content. A tablespoon of salt is equivalent to 2,325mg of sodium. The average person takes in 3,500mg per day. That is 1,200mg more than the standard DASH Effect plan and 2,000mg more than the lower sodium DASH plan. Preparing your meals with herbs and seasoning that have no added sodium will greatly reduce your sodium intake and aid in reducing those numbers drastically.

If your body has less sodium in it, your blood pressure drops, you start to feel better, and you can reduce your systolic blood pressure, giving you a better chance of not having a heart attack. A heart attack is one of the leading causes of death in the United States. Hypertension or high blood pressure is found in an average of 50 million people who have adhered to the American diet. That makes it about 1 billion people all over the world who are dealing with hypertension. That is why the DASH effect diet is recommended for all.

By eating foods high in potassium, magnesium, and calcium, we are lowering our blood pressure. The DASH effect is a dietary pattern, rather than a single nutrient diet, that's rich in antioxidants. It provides alternatives to junk food and eliminates the need for processed foods. By following a diet plan where you lower your sodium intake but increase your consumption of potassium, you are getting full and staying full longer allowing for fewer intakes of calories per day.

With the DASH effect diet plan, you will surely have a healthier body, and you will reduce your need for medication to control your blood pressure. It has also been shown that people who have participated in the studies exhibited signs of reduced depression. If we are happy with our health, we tend to be happier with our lives. By healing our bodies, we can heal our minds and feel like we can take on whatever life throws at us. So how do we follow this diet in our daily meal prep?

One way to follow this amazing diet plan is to ensure you have plenty of variety on the plate, you must have fruits, vegetables, and non-fat to low-fat dairy. With each meal, you should have two side dishes of vegetables and fruit-based desserts instead of desserts rich in sugar. You are eliminating the need for artificial sugars and processed foods. Reading labels before buying food helps us ensure we are buying the right ingredients and nutritional needs. We will discuss what we truly need later on in this book. For now, just know that reading labels and buying more fresh or frozen food options is our best way to ensure we are following the recommended food list.

In a typical DASH Effect daily meal plan, our nutritional values can look like this:

- Calories 2015
- Total fat 70g
- Saturated fat 10g
- Trans fat 0g
- Monounsaturated fat 25g
- Potassium 3,274mg
- Calcium 1,298mg
- Cholesterol 70 mg
- Sodium 1,607mg
- Total Carbohydrates 267g
- Dietary fiber 39g
- Total sugar 109g
- Protein 90g
- Magnesium 394mg

As you can see, the amount of sodium, sugar, saturated fat, and trans fat is reduced while the amount of potassium, magnesium, and calcium is increased, providing a better diet rich in nutrients. This is how we can lower our blood pressure, decrease our blood sugar, enhance the functions of our kidney, so we can feel healthier, alert, and energized.

Chapter 2: The Key Concepts Behind the DASH Effect

The DASH effect diet is a therapeutic approach to eating healthier. It helps you manage your weight, your blood pressure, your insulin sensitivity, and your blood cholesterol. What really makes the DASH effect diet great is that it not only lowers the blood pressure but it also, over time, helps you reduce your reliance on chemical substances. It is recommended for everyone from children to seniors who are trying to live healthy as much as possible. Not only does it provide health benefits, but it also has added benefit of helping you lose weight. There are no expensive supplements or shakes to purchase, making it a budget-friendly option for people who have limited funds. By eliminating processed foods, high sodium foods, all the fat in dairy, and lowering your intake of red meats, it also provides you with a low-sodium meal plan that will drastically reduce your risks of being afflicted with heart disease and cancer as well as diabetes and depression.

As with any diet or meal prep plan, there are key factors that determine why we need to change our eating habits. Whether it is high blood pressure or finding a healthier weight loss program, changing your dietary intake is hard. We don't make decisions to change our eating habits because we are told to by our doctors, it's not because the hottest stars are doing it, and it's not because we see our best friend or others online getting healthier either. It's because you are dealing with illness and want a better way to handle it, it is because you are ready to change your life and health.

When you get to the point that you have had enough of the pain, enough of the suffering from high blood pressure, enough of multiple prescriptions and are ready to make a difference in your life and your family's lives, that is when we start thinking about changing. By adding the DASH effect diet to our meal prep plans, we can start making those changes with minimal discomfort or inconvenience.

One thing we must be prepared to do is accepting that we no longer need the sodium and that food will taste good without it. Just give it time. After you eliminate all the sodium you have been adding to your meals, you will start to feel better, and your health will improve. You will notice that the taste of food has changed, and you will be able to taste more of the food and less of the sodium. Once you start the elimination process, you may feel as if your food has lost its flavor, but it hasn't. That is just the sodium leaving your body. Your taste buds will adjust themselves. Over time, you will start to taste the food, and you will have a deeper understanding of how your food should taste. You will have less of a craving for sodium, and you will even be able to tell if extra sodium was added to your food.

The key factor to making this change, and sticking with it, is to gradually reduce your sodium. Start with buying foods with low-sodium content and only sprinkling salt on the food while it cooks. Use a specific measurement and don't add any more after it is done. Gradually eliminate this habit of sprinkling salt and get used to the natural sodium that's in your food. As you decrease your sodium intake, you will notice your taste buds adjusting, and you will no longer need the sodium that you used to put on your food. The same goes for sugar and other things that you need to adjust to this diet.

By adding more fruit and vegetables to your meals, you are essentially getting those natural sugars that are necessary for your dietary and nutritional needs. Everything we eat has natural sugars, as young children we learn that sugar is good. However, we are not told that sugar can be found naturally in fruits and vegetables. As we get older, we struggle to let go of the sugars that we have added to our diet. Those sugars cause fat to build up in our bodies and can result in a higher risk of diabetes. Salt and sugar are among the hardest things to let go of, but it can happen.

If we eat healthier, we become healthier and more energized. Sugar and salt weigh us down and even make us look bloated. This can make us less energized and uncomfortable in our clothes. It increases our heart rate and changes the chemistry in our bodies. When we become healthier, our moods change, we can think better, and we won't have as many health issues. These are the key concepts behind the DASH effect diet plan.

Dietary recommendations with nutritional facts

A few dietary recommendations can make a world of difference as we transition to a new meal prep plan. What you should start with is some general knowledge about what nutrients are found in our foods. For example, fruits are low fast-food items with low sodium and lower cholesterol. This makes them a great source of vitamin C, folic acid, and dietary fiber. Fruits that are high in potassium are bananas, cantaloupe, dried apricots, and orange juice. Dietary fiber is found in fruits and can help reduce heart disease and helps with fiber intake which aids in bowel functions. Whole fruits contain enough dietary fiber to make you feel full, so you will only require a minimum amount of calories. Vitamin C helps repair body tissue and is necessary to maintain healthy teeth and gums.

Several vegetables have zero sodium content. Asparagus is one of these vegetables. If you add 5 spears of asparagus to a meal, that's enough to significantly reduce your sodium intake. Other zero-sodium vegetables are ⅓ portion of a medium cucumber, ¾ cups of green snap peas, ½ medium summer squash and 1 medium sweet corn ear. Try incorporating these into your meal prep plans. Every meal should have 1-2 vegetables. So think about adding in several more choices to your dinner plate.

Tilapia, tuna, salmon, catfish, and halibut all have low-sodium content. With a serving size of 3 ounces, you can incorporate either one of these fish into just about every meal. For example, you can have poached salmon and eggs for breakfast. Add in a cup of decaffeinated coffee and a slice of whole-wheat bread with light margarine and a medium apple, and you have yourself a very hearty breakfast with low sodium and a minimal number of processed foods. In this chapter, I have included several recipes and nutritional facts to help you start the DASH effect diet on your own.

The dietary needs of everyone and every age is different so following the standard 2000 calorie diet may not be the ideal diet plan for everyone. So I have included a dietary recommendation for women and men based on age groups below.

Age (Women)	Sedentary lifestyle	Moderate lifestyle	Active lifestyle
19-30	2000	2000-2200	2400
31-50	1800	2000	2200
51+	1600	1800	2000-2200
Age (Men)			
19-30	2400	2600-2800	3000
31-50	2200	2400-2600	2800-3000

51+	2000	2200-2400	2400-2800

Using these dietary daily nutritional values, we can then design a meal plan that incorporates these needs into the total calorie intake for the day. Below are a few recipes for meal prep items that can be used with fruit, grain, low-fat dairy, meat, and nuts or seeds of your choice. I started with a couple of breakfast recipes then provided you with a couple of lunch recipes as well as a couple of dinner recipes. Each recipe is designed to follow the DASH effect diet and is just a piece of the menu. You will notice that I have included alternatives to traditional flour as well as a vegan alternative for those who do not eat meats. Each recipe also indicates the nutritional value. Some of these recipes provide recommended toppings or garnish, and some of them are great to bring along to work as a snack or lunch.

Recipes for breakfast

Banana Pancakes

If you love bananas, then you are going to love these pancakes. This recipe should make about 4-6 pancakes and takes roughly 30-40 minutes to prepare.

Nutrition per serving:
      Calories 146
      Fat 4g
      Carbohydrates 22g
      Protein 7g
    Sodium 331g

What to use:
      Low-fat milk or lactose-free milk (0.33
      cup) Chopped walnuts (1 tablespoon)
      Vanilla extract (0.50 teaspoon)
      Olive oil (1.50 teaspoon)
      Cinnamon (A small pinch)
      Salt (A small pinch)
    Large Eggs (2)
    Baking powder (1.0 teaspoon)
      Whole-wheat flour or coconut flour (0.33
      cup) Mashed Banana (1)

What to do:
1. In a mixing bowl, combine all of the dry ingredients.
2. Separate the two eggs but keep the egg whites

3. In another mixing bowl, add olive oil, low-fat milk, egg whites, mashed banana, and vanilla until it's blended together well.
4. Combine the dry ingredients with the liquid ingredients. Using a spoon, stir until it's smooth.
5. Heat a griddle or frying pan over medium heat and apply a lite coating of olive oil to prevent the mixture from sticking. Place ¼ cup of the pancake mixture into a pan.
6. When you see bubbles around the edges of the pancakes, flip them over and continue cooking until the other side is done.
7. Sprinkle the chopped walnuts on top for added protein and texture.

Toppings:
Sugar-free syrup
Non-fat vanilla yogurt

Homemade Granola

This recipe takes 10 minutes to prepare, 30 minutes to cook, and makes 16 servings.

Nutrition per serving:
>Calories 199
>Fat 13g
>Sodium 86mg
>Carbohydrates 16g
>Protein 5g

What to use:
>Olive oil or Coconut oil (0.33 cup) Honey or Maple Syrup (0.33 cup) Salt (0.50 teaspoon)
>Cinnamon (2 Teaspoons)
>Protein Powder (0.50 cup)
>Flaxseed meal (0.50 cup)
>Raw pumpkin seeds (0.50 cup) Chopped walnuts (1 cup)
>Oats (2 cups)

What to do:
1. Start with preheating your oven to 325 °F.
2. Combine oats, walnuts, pumpkin seeds, flax, protein powder, cinnamon, and salt in a large mixing bowl.
3. Once everything is mixed well, drizzle with honey and then olive oil.
4. Stir until the mixture is evenly coated with both.
5. Prepare a baking sheet with wax paper.
6. Spread the mixture over the wax paper.
7. Continue to bake at 325°F for 30 minutes until golden brown.
8. Once done remove the granola from the stove and let it cool in the fridge for 2 hours.

Recipes for lunch

Spicy Peanut Tofu, Rice, and Avocado Salad

This recipe needs about 15 minutes to prepare. Serving size of 2 entrée sized salads.

Nutrition per serving:

      Calories 380 kcal
      Fat 18g
      Carbohydrates 42g
      Protein 15g
   Iron 14%
      Calcium 16%
      Vitamin A 15%
      Vitamin C 12%

What to use:

Dressing:

      Cayenne pepper (3-4 Dashes)
      Tamari (2 teaspoons)
   Water (0.50 cup)
      Agave syrup or Maple syrup (2 teaspoons)
      White miso paste (1 tablespoon)
   Peanut butter (2 tablespoons)

Salad:

   Mixed Spring greens (5 cups)
      Avocado, sliced-lengthwise (0.50 cups)
      Firm tofu, chilled and cubed (0.50 cup)
      Cooked brown rice (1 cup)

Garnish:

      Chopped cilantro
      Chopped peanuts
   Pepper or cayenne sprinkled on top (dash)

What to do:

1. Prepare your food processor or Vitamix.
2. Combine all the ingredients for the dressing in the food processor or Vitamix.
3. Blend until it's smooth and adjust the peanut butter as needed to get the richness of the sauce you wish for.
4. Prepare a pot with water and a pinch of salt. Once boiled, add the rice.
5. Cook rice until tender and done.
6. On a cutting board, dice up your tofu.
7. Toss your tofu in with the rice.
8. Add in a few spoonfuls of peanut sauce then proceed to toss the salad.
9. Place greens in a serving bowl.
10. Place sliced avocado over the top of the greens.
11. Decorating in a twirl design.

12. Place a scoop of the peanut tofu on top of the salad.
13. Add more dressing as needed, plus the cilantro and peanuts, cayenne pepper.

Poppy Seed Chicken Noodle Casserole

This is a twist on the classic chicken casserole. It takes 50 minutes to bake chicken and up to 2 hours once it's placed in the slow cooker. Serving size is 4.

Nutrition per serving:
> Calories 411.3
> Total Fat 8.1 g
> Cholesterol 68.4 mg
> Sodium 251.8 mg
> Carbohydrates 47.4 g
> Protein 38.7 g

What to use:
> Light buttery spread (4 tablespoons)
> Poppy seed (2 Teaspoons)
> Frozen peas (2 cups Thawed)
> Whole-wheat pasta (4 cups)
> Boneless and skinless chicken breast (2)

What to do:
1. Preheat oven to 325 °F.
2. Once it's preheated, place the chicken in a pan and cook.
3. While cooking chicken, cook the pasta until it's tender.
4. Once the pasta is done, place it in the slow cooker on low temperature.
5. Add the peas.
6. Add the poppy seeds.
7. Add the buttery spread.
8. Once the chicken is done, add it too.
9. Cook in the slow cooker until the peas are warm or for 30 minutes minimum or 2 hours maximum.
10. Season to taste.

Recipes for dinner

Easy Sweet Potato Veggie Burgers, with Avocado

This is a vegan twist on the traditional burger. Who says burgers can't be vegan? This recipe makes 6-8 burgers and takes 10 minutes to prepare and 80 minutes to cook.

Nutrition per serving:
> Total carbohydrates: 30g
> Protein: 7g

Fat: 4g
Calories: 176g
Dietary fiber: 5g

What to use:

> Chopped greens (kale, spinach, parsley) (0.33-1 cup finely)
> Nutritional yeast or any flour (try oat flour) (0.33 cup)
> Black pepper (add more for more bite!) (0.25
> teaspoon) Salt (0.50 teaspoon)
> Chipotle powder or Cajun spice (use more for spicier burgers, (0.50 -1
> teaspoon)
> Garlic powder (1 teaspoon)
> Apple cider vinegar (0.75
> teaspoon) Tahini (2-3 tablespoons)
> White onion, chopped (0.50 cup)
> Cooked white beans (canned, drained and rinsed) (16 ounces)
> Sweet potato, baked and peeled (1 medium)

Toppings:

> Avocado, tomato, Vegenaise, burger buns,
> greens *Skillet:*
> Virgin coconut oil (1 tablespoon)

Optional:

> Panko breadcrumbs for crispy coating

What to do:
1. Preheat oven to 400 °F.
2. Bake the potato for 40-60 minutes or until tender.
3. Combine potato and beans in a large mixing bowl. Beans must be rinsed before you add it to the bowl.
4. Using fork or masher, mash together the ingredients in the bowl.
5. Put in the white onions and keep mashing.
6. Put in the tahini, garlic, chipotle, salt and pepper, yeast, greens, and apple cider vinegar.
7. Keep on mashing until it's thoroughly mashed.
8. With the oven at 400 °F, heat a skillet on the stovetop over high heat and add the coconut oil.
9. Form burger patties and roll in panko crumbs if using them then place on the skillet to cook.
10. Cooking time is 1-3 minutes per side, cook patties until light brown.
11. Then repeat with all the rest of the patties, making around 6-8 patties.
12. Once all the patties are cooked, place them on a baking sheet lined with wax paper and bake for 10-15 minutes, cooking all the way through.
13. While baking the burgers, slice up your toppings for decorating the burgers.

14. Toast your whole-wheat bun in a toaster (any whole-wheat, high-fiber bun will work).
15. Add vegan mayonnaise and spicy mustard to the bun
16. When burgers are done add burger to bun and the top with your choice of toppings.
17. Serve warm!

Note: You can store the remaining burgers in a sealed container in the fridge for a day or freezer for a week. You just have to reheat it at 400 °F for about 12 minutes.

Easy Roasted Salmon

This is part of a dinner dish that includes roasted salmon. Also, you will add vegetables and fruit along with some grain. This recipe takes 10 minutes to prepare and 22 minutes to cook. Serving size of 4.

Nutrition per serving:
> Sodium 78 mg
> Calories 251
> Potassium 894 mg
> Calcium 36 mg
> Cholesterol 94 mg
> Carbohydrates 2 g
> Fat 11g
> Magnesium 53 mg
> Saturated Fat 2g
> Dietary Fiber less than 1 g
> Sugars less than 1 g
> Protein 34g

What to use:
> Garlic cloves, minced and peeled
> (4) Fresh ground pepper
> Lemon, cut (4 wedges)
> Minced fresh dill, from one small bunch (0.25 cup)
> Wild salmon fillets (4-6 ounce pieces)

What to do:
1. Preheat oven to 400 °F before starting.
2. Bring out a glass baking dish and coat it with coconut oil.
3. Place your salmon fillets in the dish.
4. Using the 4 wedges of lemon, squeeze one per fillet on top of the fillets.
5. Then sprinkle black pepper, garlic, and dill on each fillet.
6. Bake for 20-22 minutes until the fillets are opaque in the center.

Chocolate Banana Cake

This is a blend of chocolate and banana which blends really well with the cake texture. The preparation time is about 15 minutes and cooking time is around 25 minutes. This recipe can make around 18 servings.

Nutrition per serving:

Calories: 150
Sodium: 52 milligrams
Potassium: 119 milligrams
Magnesium: 19 milligrams

What to use:

Large egg (1)
    Canola oil (0.25 cup)
    Soy milk (0.75 cup)
    Ripe banana, mashed (1 large, 0.50 cup)
    Baking soda (0.50 teaspoon)
    Splenda brown sugar blend (0.50 cup)
    Unsweetened cocoa powder (0.25 cup)
    Semisweet dark chocolate chips (0.50 cup)
    All-purpose flour (2 cups)
    Vanilla extract (1 teaspoon)
    Egg white (1)
Lemon juice (1 tablespoon)

What to do:

1. Preheat your oven to 350 °F.
2. Using olive oil, coat a nonstick brownie pan.
3. Add flour to a bowl.
4. Blend in the brown sugar.
5. Cocoa and baking soda.
6. In a separate bowl throw in the bananas.
7. While whisking, pour in the soy milk, oil, eggs, egg whites, lemon juice, and the vanilla.
8. Once everything is blended, make a cavity in the flour and slowly pour in the liquid mix.
9. Add the chocolate chips.
10. Using a wooden spoon, stir to blend the ingredients.
11. Once it's thoroughly blended, spoon mixture into a brownie pan.
12. Bake for 25 minutes.
13. Take it out and use a toothpick to check the center if it is cooked all the way through.

Chapter 3: Why We Need the DASH Effect to Stay in Peak Form

Now that you know a little bit more about the DASH effect diet and how it helps your body become healthier, let's discuss why you need the DASH effect and how the myths and negative misconceptions should not be an issue once you're on this meal plan.

As we grow up, our diets get discombobulated, and we start consuming too many fried foods, too much fat, heavy creams, and way more sugar and sodium than we should have ever consumed. There is no clear-cut reason why we do this. As we age, we start trying new things, and we find an easier way to prepare meals, and we all too often take the lazy choice of stopping at the local McDonald's. Through years of eating unhealthy foods, we developed high blood pressure, insulin spikes, heart conditions, diabetes, and even depression.

We don't consider that our diet is the main cause, so we go to the doctor and get medicine that is designed with chemicals, similar to the processed foods that we have been consuming for years. The medicines help, but they do not eliminate the problem, in fact, they increase our need to be dependent on chemical-based foods and medicine. So what do we do about it? We continue to eat the garbage that is killing us, and we wonder why we aren't getting any better.

This is a cycle of self-destruction that we have carried from the early stages of life where we learned our eating habits and developed a taste for food. The DASH effect diet is against what we know as the normal way to enjoy our foods. It scares people to think that lower sodium could actually transform their health. If you are anything like the average American, you probably didn't realize the amount of sodium that is in your standard everyday diet.

That is why the DASH effect diet is the ideal way to get your health back on track. We don't need added salt in our foods. We don't need to consume 66 pounds of sugar per year. We definitely don't need to be dependent on chemical-based food and drinks. So how do we change this? We follow the DASH effect diet.

If you have been following me up until now, then you know that there are many benefits you can gain from following the DASH effect diet, and you are probably considering changing your eating habits. Maybe you're a little hesitant about eliminating the sugar and salt in your diet. You probably think that your food will not taste as good. Maybe you have tried other diets in the past, but you always ended up falling back on your old eating patterns.

Well, the good thing about the DASH effect diet is that it isn't like any other diet on the market. That is because it isn't a diet plan at all. It is a complete change in your eating patterns. But you don't have to actually change much of what you are already doing. It's mostly about portion control and buying cleaner and fresher ingredients.

If you are part of the meat-eating community that consumes 52.2 million pounds of meat per year, then it may be a bit difficult to alter your meat options for a while. In the DASH effect plan, you eat less red meat and more poultry, fish, and turkey. These are leaner meats with less fat and cholesterol. They also have a lower sodium content than pork and beef. If you are not a meat eater, then this diet will be an easy change for you. Many of the recipes that are available on the DASH effect diet are not only dairy-free but meat-free as well, making this a vegan-friendly diet.

Every year more and more people are being diagnosed with hypertension, diabetes, and heart disease. With the alarming numbers of people who suffer with these disorders, we need to consider why no one has changed their diet plan. Maybe it is out of fear of losing control over their food options. Maybe it is just because of plain stubborn behavior. Whatever the reason may be, Americans are not changing their eating patterns, it is clear that continuing the cycle of fat, deep fried, high-sodium meals are not doing any wonders for their health. The DASH effect is recommended not only by one scientist but by several companies and agencies who fight for a healthier America.

Why should you transition to the DASH effect diet? The answer: because it simply works. It's that simple and that easy. Scientifically, it has been proven to work. If something works as well as this does, it's a surprise that the school systems are not incorporating it into their weekly meal prepping for students.

How the benefits outweigh any myths or negative press on the effects

So why hasn't it taken off? There is a long-running myth that fresh foods are not as cheap as processed foods. But this simply isn't true. The process of preparing fresher foods that are richer in vitamins and nutrients and contain less fat-burning calories means that you will need a lower intake of calories and that your food will keep you full longer, essentially costing less in the long run.

People often believe that going to the drive-thru at McDonald's or Burger King is easier than preparing a kale salad. After a long day at work, you don't feel like coming home to prepare a healthy meal. It takes longer, and you just don't have the time or energy. This too is not true. It takes about 15 minutes to prepare a meal acceptable for the DASH effect diet, once all the prep work has been completed. You can also prepackage your ingredients or practice food prep procedures by preparing your ingredients before work and placing them in a slow cooker to simmer all day. This allows for you to simply come home, grab a bowl, and relax on the couch or at the table with family while enjoying a healthy, clean, and fresh meal.

Many people believe that there is a learning curve to proper nutritional calorie intake food prep. This as well is not true. There are so many recipes and cookbooks on the market that are geared towards healthier and cleaner eating that you'll find a recipe in no time to prepare for dinner. The best part is whatever you have left over from dinner can be utilized for breakfast or even lunch depending on what it is. Many of our food options on the DASH effect diet plan can be used for multiple meals, such as apples can be used as breakfast, fruit side dishes, and even desserts. Often times, people think that eating healthy means eating bland food. That simply isn't true. Just because it's healthy doesn't make it bland. There are so many reasons why this myth is present, one of them being that throughout our life we have added salt and sugar to everything we eat, chose the fattest parts of the meat, and excessively flavored our foods. We do this because we are conditioned into thinking that we must add flavor to food. However, food already has a flavor. The natural juices and flavors that are ingrained in the fruit and vegetables provide all the flavor you need for your meal to taste amazing.

Now that doesn't mean that adding herbs to your food isn't a good thing. Many herbs and nectars provide healing benefits that just can't be ignored. Rosemary helps with immunity and honey is an antihistamine. Garlic is good for reducing blood pressure as well as combating the common cold. Sage is known for its anti-inflammatory properties as well as antioxidants. As you can see, many herbs and nectars provide added benefits to your food. So the best rule of thumb is to taste the natural foods then add in a few flavors through fresh herbs to give it an added health benefit.

Herbs can be purchased dried as well as fresh. Many people believe the benefits of herbs are just as effective when dried. I find that fresh herbs give a much better aromatic smell and tend to have a fresher, cleaner taste. They blend better with our foods and gives that added touch of texture that you just can't get from powders or dried herbs. They also are not processed heavily and have not been mixed with added sodium and other chemicals to make them last longer. As with any fresh food, being frozen is the best route since they still retain all the nutrients that provide you with the healthiest caloric intake.

Many Americans have been buying processed and canned foods since World War 2. They are marketed as containing all the health benefits of a fresh batch of vegetables. However, through the process of canning or processing at the factory, we have learned that they are missing key components to their nutritional value. So the myth that canned or processed foods are just as good as fresh is completely wrong. Not only are they higher in sodium, since it is added for flavor and sustainability. But they are having their key nutrients flash steamed or cooked out of them and then being mixed with sustainable chemicals to make them last longer on the shelf. Taking all this into account, we should always purchase our foods frozen or fresh to ensure we are feeding ourselves and our families the best possible combination of nutrients that we can afford. One way we can do this is through farmers' markets and at local farms.

Buying your food at a farmers' market or picking your own at a local farm can also reduce the cost of the food you are purchasing. Knowing what you want to prepare in advance is also a way of reducing your cost of groceries, and it will also provide you with a guideline to decide on what kind of meal you should cook each day. This allows you to prepare your ingredients in advance and be ready for mealtime without the extra hassle. It doesn't take a ton of extra time to learn how to prepare in advance. You simply need to know what you like and have a recipe or idea of how you want to prepare a meal once you're ready for meal prep time. This will cut down on the amount of time it takes to prepare the meal without adding extra time to your daily to-do list. Later in this book, we will lay out a method to meal prep with a list of options for each meal and a way to incorporate an accountability partner into your diet change.

Chapter 4: Who Should Not Use the DASH Effect and Why?

Previously, we discussed who the DASH Effect diet is ideal for. As rated by the Food and Drug Administration the DASH Effect diet is rated safe for everyone. So who shouldn't use the DASH effect diet then? Well, that is simple, this diet is not for people that are not committed to making a positive change in their lives. If you do not want to be healthier, if you do not want to lose weight, if you enjoy having diabetes and hypertension, if you do not want to transform your health and make changes to your lifestyle that will reduce your blood pressure, help you lose weight and also feel more happy in general about life, then you should not use the DASH effect diet.

Who in your family does this sound like? Is this person you? Or is it someone else that has been using their disease as a reason to play the victim every day of their life? You see the DASH effect diet is not for quitters. It's not for those people who love having sickness and struggle to keep up with their children or grandchildren. It is not for those that would rather eat a high-sodium and high-sugar diet. It is definitely not for those people who think that if their food is not loaded with bacon grease, it's not good.

In today's families, we all have that one person that doesn't watch what they eat. They think food doesn't determine their health, or they just really don't care. That person is not the ideal person to try the DASH effect diet. Not because they don't need it, not because it wouldn't help them, and definitely not because they are immune to its benefits or allergic to the process. No, those people are not ideal for the DASH effect diet because they do not care how they are treating their bodies. They don't care if they have ailments that they can reduce and eliminate. The simply do not care about the state of their health.

So how do you help those who don't care? We all would know they need the DASH effect diet and that if they were to give it a try, they would not only be happier, but they will also see drastic changes in their health for the better. So instead of shoving the DASH effect diet down their throats and trying to force them to get healthy, we must first get healthy ourselves. The best way to lead someone to a better path for their life is to show them through your own actions that it works and to essentially trigger their jealousy, so they want to get healthy to spite you.

Now I know this sounds a bit petty and far-fetched, but isn't it true that sometimes you only wanted something simply because someone else had it? Exactly, so now you see where this chapter is going. So far we have discussed what the DASH effect diet is, whom it's suited for, why it is effective, and now we will discuss the positive effects it has on our mental psyche.

Have you ever done something that you thought you were going to fail at, but in the end you actually did not fail? What about winning an award for something you did inadvertently while doing something else? Well, that feeling you got when that award was won, or that amazing realization that you actually succeeded instead of failing is what the DASH effect diet does for your psyche. Imagine going in for a haircut and coming out with a stylish haircut, a new dye job, and some free hair-conditioning supplies.

When you get so focused on creating a healthy eating habit you forget about so many other things that you are accomplishing. Such as losing weight or lowering your insulin injection needs. What if we could all just wake up with no depression, no diseases, no cancers, and no excess fat? With the DASH effect diet, we eventually can. Now, do you still want to question the validity of the DASH effects?

To get healthy and reduce your blood pressure you have to start somewhere, and the DASH effect diet is exactly where you need to start. Do not be disappointed if you have setbacks because they are normal. As long as you figure out the triggers and do what you can to avoid them you should be able to continue the program without too many setbacks.

But what if my blood pressure isn't elevated? Well, then the DASH effect diet is still the best for you. It is a starting point for a healthier and cleaner lifestyle. No, I don't mean cleaner like you cleaned your house. By saying cleaner, I mean that your food comes from the ground, with no pesticides, no growth hormones, no chemicals, and no processing.

What else do you need to know to understand that the DASH effect diet is for everyone? All it takes to find out if it is for you, besides me telling you it is, is to get started today. In this book, I have provided you a detailed description of what the DASH effect is and how to incorporate it into your life. But one thing we haven't talked about yet is the motivation you need to bring about changes in your life with the DASH effect. That is what this whole chapter will be on, motivational techniques to keep you focused, to keep you moving forward, and to show those stubborn family members who think that food does not heal, that in fact, it does.

One proven method to motivate you to continue on your journey with the DASH effect diet is to see progress. Progress is wonderful. It's like a reward in itself. When you see that your blood pressure is lower or you are experiencing less blood sugar spikes for example. That is called progress. Maybe your doctor has noticed a positive change in your blood. Maybe when you stand in front of the mirror after your shower, you see a slimmer and healthier you. Progress can be anything from a slight change in the size of your pants to a drastic drop in your need for your blood pressure medication. Whatever progress you achieved, regardless of how small it is, you need to celebrate.

Celebrate in ways that don't undermine your progress. There are many ways to celebrate your progress without having to derail your new lifestyle. One of my favorite ways to celebrate a positive change in my life is to immediately give myself praise. I look myself in the mirror, and I tell myself all the things that are wonderful about what I have accomplished. I acknowledge the efforts I have made, and I congratulate myself on a job well done. This is a personalized pat on the back.

Another way to reward yourself is to buy yourself a new piece of clothing, something that fits your new waistline. This tells your mind that you are making changes to get a more beneficial lifestyle. It also gives you a wonderful endorphin boost when you look at that new, slim piece of clothing and think, "I did this." Just remember that you are working towards a healthier you and that healthier 'you' will need a whole new wardrobe eventually. By throwing away clothes that no longer fit, you are subconsciously telling your mind and body that you will no longer accept what your body was back then. This is like a confirmation that you are a new person. Buying new clothes helps us physically see the changes we are making, giving us a good reason to celebrate our accomplishments and progress while making sure we look amazing.

Accountability is another great way to reward yourself when you see great progress. Accountability is when someone else will hold you accountable for your goals. This will be discussed later in Chapter 6, but for now, we will just state that accountability is calling your friend, your mom, or your exercise buddy and celebrating with them about your progress. Remember they are on your side and know that you need this healthier lifestyle.

There are so many ways to celebrate your achievements. By setting goals and reaching them, you are rewarding yourself every day when you pick healthier options and become a healthier you. Sometimes just knowing is enough of a reward. However, if knowing that you are getting healthier isn't enough, you can always try a day at the spa, a movie with your best friend, or even a night out with your favorite girl/guy.

One of the best rewards you can give yourself is acknowledging that you have done it on your own, without medicines, without surgeries, and without sitting around thinking there is nothing you can do to get healthier. You are the deciding factor, and you made that one decision to make your life better. Whatever you choose as a reward, make sure it is something that will give you excitement and that feeling of accomplishment. When we don't feel like we accomplished something big, we tend to feel more sad than happy. The trick is to be excited about your progress even if it seems insignificant.

Chapter 5: Specific Benefits to Your Health Gained from the DASH Effect

Since you made it this far, you have heard over and over that the DASH effect has outstanding scientific evidence showing its validity and the effects it has on your health. So what more can I say to motivate you on getting started with the DASH effect diet? Maybe with the amazing effects the DASH diet can have on our health, we will see a potential for lower insurance rates. Not only are our insurance rates on the verge of dropping because of this amazing diet, but it's also a national dietary method that's been recommended for over 10 years. Another benefit to the DASH effect diet is that previous studies proved that staying on the DASH effect diet can result in a reduction of systolic and diastolic blood pressure. These results were across all age groups, races, and genders. That means that this diet works for all races.

We all know that many African Americans suffer from race-specific anomalies and that these anomalies can cause certain diseases to be more dominant and prevalent. One thing scientists learned in the trials was that this diet worked amazingly on the African American community as well as the Caucasians, Asians, and Indians.

Further findings revealed that the DASH effect diet also lowered the risk of stroke and coronary heart disease, making it beneficial for people who are afflicted with such conditions. The DASH effect diet has also helped with bone loss and density, reducing bone turnover, which means an improvement in bone health for those prone to osteoporosis.

There are many ways for the DASH effect diet to help you with weight loss. Below are just a few of the ways:

Fruits and veggies are low in calories.

They are more filling as well

You include protein-rich foods in every meal

Using protein for snacks can increase your
energy Protein makes meals more satisfying

Protein also helps with in-between blood sugar crashes

By focusing on the healthy foods, you eliminate the need for junk
foods By eating denser foods, you reduce your cravings

You can make the DASH effect diet your lifestyle diet plan

It's not a fad diet

Carbohydrates are not used to fill you up

The plan doesn't limit your protein

There is less starch

Protein supports muscle mass

Proteins are energy boosters and provide us the energy to exercise more
efficiently

High blood pressure is a big reason why the DASH effect is popular. By reducing your sodium intake, you end up reducing your blood pressure. There are a few other benefits that we haven't discussed throughout this book:

It helps reduce your blood pressure by reducing sodium in your diet

It also helps by reducing your weight which can raise your blood pressure

By reducing your weight and raising your protein intake you have more
energy

More energy means you can exercise more and help lower your blood
pressure

The DASH effect diet provides a healthy eating plan that not only reduces
your blood pressure but helps keep it stabilized

We all know that high blood pressure increases the risk of getting heart disease and can contribute to several other diseases and ailments. The DASH effect can help eliminate the chances of heart disease by lowering your blood pressure. Several of the benefits of the DASH effect have been discussed throughout this book and in this chapter. But there are more benefits that the DASH effect can provide to aid in lowering the risk of heart disease:

By adding more fiber, calcium, and magnesium, you can reduce the risk
of heart disease

Those three minerals help regulate blood
pressure Potassium stops the effects of sodium

The DASH effect diet is a sustainable diet, it is not something that will end immediately

It's low in sodium and high in nutrient-rich foods

It is adaptable, low stress, and easily customizable, making it the best diet choice for all

Even with all the benefits that the DASH effect diet has been proven to have on your health, not many people are using it. Though it has changed the way people think about eating and how food can transform your health, people are still so reluctant to what they have considered as proper eating their whole life. So why are more people not using the DASH effect diet? This is partly because the patients who need the diet the most are only getting medicinal help from their primary care providers. Not many doctors have nutritional backgrounds and lack knowledge in this area. Perhaps many people can be helped immensely if part of a doctor's training included nutrition and diet plans.

Although doctors are not trained to properly help those dealing with a diet issue, nutritionists are, and there are many ways you can get in contact with one. Health coaches are trained to help you find the right diet plan for your needs. Some of them should be listed in your local online business directory. Finding the right coach to help you with the DASH effect diet will take some time. Try asking family and friends. Get opinions online from trusted friends. Research the options in your area and know exactly what you are looking for.

Even with all the research and referrals, you still won't be able to know if that coach is right for you until you have a face-to-face meeting with them. So sit down with the coach of your choice and ask all the questions that you need to. Make sure you make a list of the questions you want to ask, this will ensure that you will get to know that person better. Once you run out of questions, ask the coach if there is anything else they would like to include in their comments or if they have any questions. This is a sure way to hear out your coach's opinions.

Remember they are the experts and know exactly what to do to help you with your dietary needs. One question you might ask is: "Are they familiar with the DASH effect diet?" This should instantly tell you whether or not they are the right nutritionist for you.

With all the talk about nutrition, food portions, and benefits associated with the DASH effect diet, this book would not be complete without helpful tools. These tools are designed to teach you how to incorporate proper meal preparations, exercise, accountability, and so much more. For the next chapter, we will be looking at those tools, and we will learn how to utilize them. The first tool we will look at is accountability, how you can find an accountability partner, and what you can expect from an accountability partner. You will notice that in this section we discussed nutritionists and health coaches a little bit more. That is because a health coach is a great accountability partner. Part of their roles in your life is to help you become accountable for your food choices, they act as your support system, and of course, they're your motivational coach.

The next part would deal with the subject of getting healthy with the help of exercise. We discussed various ways to incorporate exercise into your healthy lifestyle. There are many forms of exercise, and as a person with health issues, you might want to consult a doctor about appropriate exercises that you can do without endangering your health. Making sure that you are not overexerting yourself or injuring yourself is the best way to start a new exercise routine. In the next chapter, we will talk about yoga, running, jogging, and cardio. These are all acceptable exercises even for someone who has been dealing with various health concerns.

Meal prep is a big part of the DASH effect diet, and it can make or break your progress. Since you were proactive and bought this book, you have already set yourself up for success. This book not only explains the information on why this diet plan works, but it also helps you prepare the right meals so that you can take complete advantage of the DASH effect diet. Meal preparation is an easy thing to do if you use the worksheet provided in the next chapter. There is a designated section for each day and each meal. There is also a list of serving sizes and approved foods.

This is just a starting point. Once you get the hang of the process, you will find yourself creating your own meal preparation worksheets or even designing a digital one to use on the go. Meal preparation sounds like a chore, but you shouldn't feel discouraged because it can give you something to look forward to, such as that amazing meal you planned for the next day.

But meal preparations would be nothing without the calorie intake worksheet. It is designed to show you during the first few weeks of your journey into the DASH effect diet how well you are following the guidelines set by the program. By keeping track of the calories that you are taking in and making sure you stay within the recommended limits for each nutrient, you are following the program as designed. Doing what you can to meet the requirements of the DASH effect diet can help make sure that you will arrive at the desired outcome, a healthier and happier   life.

Chapter 6: Ways to Include the DASH Effect into Your Daily Meals

There is so much information about the DASH effect diet packed into this book that I'm sure it is confusing, and you are probably feeling a bit overwhelmed. But there's no need to stress yourself out. We will now talk about how you can incorporate it into your daily meals.

We all hear that breakfast is the most important meal of the day, and if you are like most Americans, you either do not have time for breakfast or you just grab something from the local donut shop or McDonald's on the way to work. If you want to adhere to the principles of the DASH effect diet, that will not do. We are looking for cleaner, healthier ways to get all the nutrients we need for the day without all the added sodium and processed foods. So when we grab a donut from the local donut shop, we are basically fueling our day from the start with sugar, and that isn't good. When you start your day with sugar by mid-morning, you will have a sugar crash and need an energy boost later on. Instead, we should start the day with protein and low-sodium, low-sugar foods.

One of the best ways to start your day would be with a granola bowl packed with nuts, fruits, oats, and honey. This sounds like a lot of work, but it's really quite easy. You can prepare this in advance and have it stored in your fridge in mason jars so you can bring it to work. There are many recipes online that you can use, and many of them have nutritional information so you can track your calorie intake. You can use the worksheet which is found later in this book.

It isn't very hard to incorporate a new eating plan into your day, it just takes a bit of conscious effort to change the way you have been doing things. It can be scary but knowing that you are doing it to improve your health is a great way to keep you motivated as you continue your transition to a healthier life.

As you try to make your diet super healthy, you will notice that you are feeling more energized, and you will feel like you want to do more exercises during the day. Later in this chapter, we will discuss exercises that you can incorporate into your lifestyle to add to the DASH effect program and help you with establishing your healthier, new life. For now, just understand that if you have been sedentary for a while or if you are not as active as you should be, it will take time, and you should start slow, so you don't burn out quickly.

Accountability is another thing that will make this journey through the DASH effect program easier. Accountability is the number one thing that people who are making changes in their life say they lack. Many people aren't sure how to acquire an accountability partner nor are they sure about what one should be doing for them. Later on, we will discuss accountability and how it can help you with your healthier lifestyle journey.

This chapter is packed full of great resources and tools that will aid you in transforming your life with the help of the DASH effect diet. To make the most out of this book and the DASH effect you definitely need to use the information in this chapter to its fullest potential. By using all of these tools, you are giving yourself a greater advantage at accomplishing your goals such as seeing your blood pressure lower and a decrease in your medical expenses.

Exercise

Exercise is an integral part of your daily needs. If you are eating healthy and not doing any exercises, then you are only doing half the work. Starting an exercise routine when you feel like you have more energy is a great way to aid in your process of lowering your blood pressure. There are many exercise programs out there, and there are plenty of ways to incorporate them into your lifestyle. What you can start with is light cardio.

Cardio is any exercise that is mild and gets your heart rate up. You can start with walking at a fast pace. If you choose walking as an exercise, you should increase your heart rate just enough that you start breathing heavily, but you should still be capable of holding a conversation without gasping for air. Gasping for air means that you are overexerting your body and no longer burning calories. If you do incorporate a cardio routine into your lifestyle, make sure you increase your calorie intake based on the chart listed in chapter 2.

If cardio is not your style, a light yoga exercise is also a great way to stretch and get that heart rate up. Starting with the beginner's yoga, you can learn the proper techniques to doing yoga and increase your body's strength and flexibility. Yoga is incredibly beneficial to your body and your mind. Not only does it provide you a mindfulness exercise, but it helps you stretch those muscles that have been weighed down by the excess fat that you have been carrying. Yoga can be practiced at home with some really great YouTube yoga teachers, or you can get a membership to a Yoga studio and get personalized help with a custom muscle test and body flexibility test. As with any exercise program consult your doctor before starting.

If those two do not sound like your cup of tea then maybe you should try jogging, running, or weightlifting. Whatever it is that you end up picking, make sure you have consulted your doctor before starting a new exercise routine. As with any new activity or change in your life, there will be some difficulties, which is why you need to stay vigilant and determined to continue with making healthy changes in your life.

Accountability

Accountability is something we hear about often. When we are at work, we are accountable for our work and the work of our teams or employees. When we go to the gym, our spotter is accountable for our lives when we exercise. As we drive down the road, we are accountable for all the pedestrians, other cars, and people in our cars to keep them safe. So the concept of accountability is nothing new.

The difference between this accountability and the others listed above is that here we are having someone else help us be accountable for making positive changes in our lives. Maybe your doctor is your accountability partner, or maybe he or she is just monitoring your changes. If you have a strong partner who can help you through the process of change, then you should know what a strong support system feels like. However, if your partner is not very helpful or you are single, then you need to find someone to help you as an accountability partner.

One of the best ways to find an accountability partner is to find someone who is willing to help you make these positive changes in your life. Talk with your friends, your family, your workout buddies, maybe even your desk mate at work. Also, your partner must change as well if they need to. If you can't find anyone in your own group or circle, then check with a nutritionist that follows the DASH effect program and sign up for accountability partner programs. You can find these online.

A health coach is someone that will help you with your food choices and teach you how to bring the DASH effect diet off the road and into restaurants. They will also help you with grocery shopping. Sometimes we need that extra help so that we don't get overwhelmed. That is where the health coach comes in. They will hold you accountable when you need that extra kick to continue on your healthy journey. As an accountability partner, you can expect them to be vigilant with your progress. They will give you tasks to complete, and they will not allow you to fail. They will also be there to celebrate with you when you accomplish wonderful things through your lifestyle change.

Celebrating your accomplishments with someone is one of the perks of having a health coach. They get to see you go through your trials and tribulations. They get to watch you succeed and see the joy you experience when you accomplish more than you ever dreamed possible. Being with a health coach or nutritionist is like having a support system with you at all times. You can do the DASH effect program without a health coach, or nutritionist, however, you cannot do it without an accountability partner. Their job is to keep you on track and then celebrate when you accomplish small victories until you reach the biggest accomplishment of your life.

An accountability partner is just that, a partner. Someone that stands with you in solidarity and supports your efforts to make positive changes in your life. If you hire a health coach, they have many useful tools to help you with your transformation while you're on the DASH effect diet. If you have an accountability partner that is just a friend or family member, their role in your journey is to support you, give you motivational pep talks, help you make proper choices, check in with you often to see how it's going, and also remind you of why you are making these changes to your lifestyle.

Meal prep worksheet

When it comes to preparing your meal plan for the week, you should pick options from this list of allowable food items. You need a specific number of servings per food group for your daily intake of calories. Listed below is the amount of each item you need with options for that food group that is acceptable.

Pick the appropriate amount from each list and then arrange them in an easy-to-follow meal plan in the sections provided for each day of the week.

Grains (7 servings per day)	Meats (2-3 servings per day)
Vegetables (5 servings per day)	Nuts (2 servings per day)
Fruit (5 servings per day)	Fats (3 servings per day)
Dairy (3 servings per day)	Sweets (2 servings per week)

Permissible foods

Apples	Asparagus
Avocado	Broccoli
Berries (strawberries, blueberries)	Bell peppers (sweet)
Cantaloupe	Carrots
Cherries	Collard greens
Cherry tomatoes	Cucumbers
Celery	Dark green lettuce (not iceberg)

Grapefruit	Hot peppers
Grapes	Eggplant
Kiwi	Kale
Lemon	Red leafy lettuce
Mangoes	Spinach
Papayas	Summer squash
Peaches	Sweet corn
Pears	Sweet potato
Pineapple	Mushrooms
Tangerines	
Watermelon	
Chicken	Brown Rice
Catfish	Cereal
Cod	Whole-grain bread
Crab	Whole-wheat pasta
Egg whites	Almonds
Halibut	Lentils
Lean ground beef	Kidney beans
Shrimp	Peas
Tuna	Sunflower seeds
Turkey	
Salmon	
Low-fat mayonnaise	Fat-free milk
Margarine (no salt added)	Low-fat milk
Olive oil	Low-fat yogurt
Low-fat baked goods	Low-fat cheese

Low-fat jelly	Coffee (decaffeinated)
Low-fat sorbet	Tea (green)
Low-fat candies	Basil
Sugar treats	Bay leaf
	Cayenne
	Chive
	Cinnamon
	Clove
	Endive
	Garlic
	Ginger
	Mint
	Parsley
	Pepper
	Rosemary
	Sage
	Turmeric

Meal prep weekly plan

Example meal prep weekly plan

Monday	Ingredients
Breakfast: Fresh mixed fruits, (1 cup) Bran muffin (1) Trans-free margarine (1 teaspoon) Fat-free milk (1 cup) Herbal tea	melons, banana, apple, and berries topped with fat-free, low-calorie vanilla-flavored yogurt (1 cup) Walnuts (0.33 cup)
Lunch: Spinach salad made with: reduced-sodium wheat crackers (12) Fat-free milk (1 cup)	Fresh spinach leaves (4 Cups) Slivered almonds (0.33 cup) Sliced pear (1) Canned mandarin orange sections (0.50 cup) Red wine vinaigrette (2 Tablespoons)
Dinner: Beef and vegetable kebab, Pecans (0.33 cup) Cooked wild rice (1 cup) Pineapple chunks (1 cup) Cran-Raspberry spritzer	**Kabob made with:** Peppers, mushrooms and onions, cherry tomatoes (1 cup each) Beef (3 ounces) Spritzer made with: sparkling water (4-8 ounces)

	Cran-Raspberry juice (4 ounces)

Monday	Ingredients
Breakfast	
Lunch	
Dinner	

Tuesday	Ingredients
Breakfast	
Lunch	
Dinner	

Wednesday	Ingredients
Breakfast	

Lunch	
Dinner	

Thursday	Ingredients
Breakfast	
Lunch	
Dinner	

Friday	Ingredients
Breakfast	
Lunch	
Dinner	

Saturday	Ingredients
Breakfast	
Lunch	
Dinner	

Sunday	Ingredients
Breakfast	
Lunch	
Dinner	

As you can see at the top of the meal preparation worksheet, I have included a sample of meal preparation. When planning meals for the day or week, it is best to put them on paper so you can see in detail exactly what you want to have and what ingredients you need. By preparing this in advance, you are taking a lot of the guesswork out of meal preparations. Earlier in the book, we discussed how knowing what you need at the grocery store helps you prepare for your meals without overspending at the grocery store. Being proactive with your meal preparations helps budget your grocery bill. For instance, when you go to the grocery store, you are not going to buy a bunch of stuff that you don't need if you already made a list of the groceries you need for the DASH effect diet program.

Each section represents a day in the week, and each block within that table is designated for meal time. Within each mealtime, you should list the name or type of meal it is, e.g. 'Slow cooked chicken.' Then on the right-hand side is the section where you list your ingredients. This will not only help in preparing the meal when the time comes, but it will also provide you with a grocery list for each week's combined meal plans. By writing this out, you are better preparing yourself for a healthier lifestyle. You can utilize this same process for every week. If you want to be a bit more proactive, you can plan your meals for several weeks out.

Some people prepare a whole meal plan for a month, as this helps them organize their weeks and days better, as well as budget their grocery shopping. By meal planning with a detailed diagram such as this one, you can make sure that you won't be eating the same meals every week as well. This gives you more options for variety in your food preparations and also allows you to see your week's meal preparation in an organized fashion, helping you eliminate the need to hunt and find something to prepare for the evening.

One thing to remember is to prepare enough that you can save your leftovers for the next day or two to save on grocery money. For instance, if you make cinnamon apples for your night time snack or if you decided on having fruit for dinner, you can blend the leftovers together and make applesauce for your morning oats tomorrow. Many of the dishes you can make for dinner can be utilized for lunch the next day, eliminating the need to prepare a designated meal plan for every single day. It also allows you to cut down on your food expenses by giving you two meals out of one grocery purchase.

If you are a single serving household, you may even get several meals out of each recipe that you make. If you prepare a meal that can serve four people, that should allow you to have lunch for the next day and dinner for the day after that. Remember, food stays fresh if it's frozen after being cooked. So, if you prepare a larger meal and only need one serving at a time, freezing the remaining portions is a great way to extend your meals for more than one day or week.

If you can squeeze in enough time, you may even prep all weekly meals in one day of the week like Sunday for example. Then you freeze them in containers and pull them out as needed. If you only need one serving of each item per meal, then you must remember to only store it in single serving sections so that you are not reheating the excess and potentially ruin the possibility of having that meal on another day. Since reheating can spoil food if it's frozen and reheated again, you should only reheat what you're going to eat.

Calorie intake tracking worksheet

For each meal you prepare, you want to keep track of the calories that you are taking in. This includes all nutritional values. This is not to keep track of calories, but it's more about keeping track of your progress with the DASH effect diet plan. This is a simple process that can easily be done by using the packaging from your food choices to record the nutritional calorie intake from the serving size suggested on the package.

If you use fresh vegetables and fruits, this can be a little bit tricky. So I am listing a few of them below so you can have a few clues as to what you would need to write down for those fresh fruits and vegetables while you're on the DASH effect diet. You can find these nutritional statistics online at the FDA website. Once you have a guideline for fresh fruits and vegetables, record that data and utilize it to meet the conditions on your calorie tracker.

Servings sizes per fruit or vegetable

A vegetable's serving size is one cup of raw mixed greens or 0.50 cup of chopped vegetables. A fruit's serving size is 1 medium fruit or a 0.50 cup of fresh, frozen, or canned fruit:

Apples

Calories 130
Potassium 260mg
    Total carbohydrates 34g
    Dietary fiber 5g
    Sugars 25g
    Proteins 1g

Bananas

Calorie 110
Potassium 450mg
    Total carbohydrates
    30g Dietary fiber 3g
    Sugars 19g
    Protein 1g

Grapes

Calories 90
Sodium 15mg
Potassium 240mg
    Total carbohydrates
    23g Dietary fiber 1g
Sugars 20g

Pineapple

Calories 50
Sodium 10mg
Potassium 120mg
    Total carbohydrates
    13g Dietary fiber 1g
Sugar 10g protein 1g

Asparagus

Calories 20

Potassium 230mg
    Total carbohydrates
    4g Dietary fiber 2g
    Sugar 2g
    Protein 2g

Carrot

Calories 30
Sodium 60mg
Potassium 250mg
    Total carbohydrates
    7g Dietary fiber 2g
    Sugars 5g
    Proteins 1g

Mushrooms

Calories 20
Sodium 15mg
Potassium 300mg
    Total carbohydrates
    3g Dietary Fiber 1g
Protein 3g

So, as you can see, you will list the nutrients that are shown here. Most of the time you will have sodium, potassium, total carbohydrates, dietary fiber, sugar, and protein on the list. These things are what you would add together to find your total intake of those nutrients. The calories section is a combined rating of these nutrients, and that is what you will need to add together to get the total daily calorie intake to meet the 2000 calories recommended by the USDA.

At the bottom of the tracker worksheets, there is an example you can utilize for your calorie tracking needs. Each meal is labeled at the top as breakfast, lunch, dinner, and snack or drink. This helps you know exactly which column to put the calories and nutrients under. The side column has listings for several of the nutrients that you want to keep track of. If you notice at the top of the chart, that is the total calories for that meal. At the end of the day, you can add all the calories together to make sure you actually had the proper intake of calories for a full day. The average calorie intake is 2,000 calories depending on your size, age, and activity level.

Calories and nutrients tracker

	Breakfast	Lunch	Dinner	Snack and

210

Nutritional Data   drinks

Monday

Calories					
Potassium					
Total Carbohydrates					
Dietary fiber					
Sugar					
Protein					
sodium					

Nutritional Data Tuesday	Breakfast	Lunch	Dinner	Snack and drinks
Calories				
Potassium				
Total Carbohydrates				
Dietary fiber				
Sugar				
Protein				
sodium				

Nutritional Data Wednesday	Breakfast	Lunch	Dinner	Snack and drinks
Calories				
Potassium				
Total Carbohydrates				
Dietary fiber				
Sugar				
Protein				
sodium				

Nutritional Data Thursday	Breakfast	Lunch	Dinner	Snack and drinks
Calories				
Potassium				
Total Carbohydrates				
Dietary fiber				
Sugar				
Protein				
sodium				

Nutritional Data Friday	Breakfast	Lunch	Dinner	Snack and drinks
Calories				
Potassium				
Total Carbohydrates				
Dietary fiber				
Sugar				
Protein				
sodium				

Nutritional Data Saturday	Breakfast	Lunch	Dinner	Snack and drinks
Calories				
Potassium				
Total Carbohydrates				
Dietary fiber				
Sugar				
Protein				
sodium				

Nutritional Data Sunday	Breakfast	Lunch	Dinner	Snack and drinks
Calories				
Potassium				
Total Carbohydrates				
Dietary fiber				
Sugar				
Protein				
sodium				

Example of the nutrition tracker

Nutritional Data Sunday	Breakfast	Lunch	Dinner	Snack and drinks
Calories	252	194	251	150
Potassium	822mg	410mg	894mg	119mg
Total Carbohydrates	33g	27g	2g	27g
Dietary fiber	8g	4g	less than 1g	1g
Sugar	8g	1g	less than 1g	9g
Protein	11g	17g	34g	3g
sodium	102mg	450mg	78mg	52mg

After a week of tracking what your calorie intake is, you will be able to see where you need to adjust your diet and how to make it less sodium-heavy and more protein, potassium, magnesium, and calcium heavy. Our health is determined by what we choose to eat. If you chose to eat fatty and greasy foods, then your body will become sluggish, tired, weak, and you might end up suffering from hypertension, diabetes, and sometimes heart conditions.

CPSIA information can be obtained
at www.ICGtesting.com
Printed in the USA
LVHW011400070121
675556LV00006B/807

9 789814 952132